People Are Saying

A well written, practical guide on a key topic for this generation. Dr. Susan deals directly and succinctly with both the myths and the realities of those factors in kids lives that affect their weight. As a pediatrician who specializes in nutrition and prevention, I will use this book to help parents of already overweight youngsters as well as those whose children are at risk but not overweight, in order to help them prevent excess weight gain.

> **—Marc S. Jacobson, MD,** Professor of Pediatrics,
> Albert Einstein College of Medicine, Director, Center for
> Atherosclerosis Prevention, Schneider Children's Hospital

Dr. Susan cuts through the confusion about what to do if your child is overweight and courageously challenges parents to take charge and make informed choices. Follow her balanced and inspiring dose of approaches and your kids will make healthy choices, even when you're not there to remind them.

> **—Barbara Glickstein, RN, MPH, MS,** Health Reporter and
> Radio Host, Martha Stewart Living Radio

Dr. Susan gives great advice to parents on how to be an educator about health, set a good example, give their children the power of choice, and be supportive This book will help parents realize that that they are the true advocates in their child's health.

> **—Shawna Rocha,** Executive Camp Director,
> Camp California Fitness

She's already guided thousands of teens toward healthier living. Now Dr. Susan teaches the parents of younger kids how to get results and make them stick.

> **—Ellis Henican,** *Newsday*

Drawing on advice from medical, health, and exercise professionals, this comprehensive handbook offers balanced suggestions that go beyond the nutritional aspects of the problem. Packed with hundreds of anecdotes from parents and kids, it offers sensible suggestions that can be implemented by any parent who wishes to see their child's health, esteem, and social life improve dramatically.

—Independent Publisher, Highlighted Titles

Parents will love this guide because Dr. Susan really gets what today's moms and dads face when it comes to establishing and maintaining healthy eating habits at home. Her realistic solutions empower families and set them up for life-long health.

—Geodie Baxter Padgett, Editor, *ParentGuide* (Florida)

Parents frequently ask me how to raise children with healthy eating habits and a positive body image. At last I can give them a tool I am confident will show them the way! Dr. Susan addresses all these issues and more, giving parents fun, effective strategies for creating a healthy child and family.

—Jen Biblowitz, LMHC, School Counselor

Dr. Susan not only educates parents on what they need to know, but gives them an easy-to-implement plan so they can get started as soon as they read the book. This is a must-read for any parent concerned about their child's weight and its affect on their health.

—Elisa Ast All, MSJ, Editor-in-Chief, iParenting Media

Trusted mother and psychologist, Dr. Susan Bartell dispels prevalent food myths, pinpoints dietary culprits and offers practical advice. By reading Bartell's wisdom, parents begin making informed nutritional decisions—and inspire healthy eating habits in children.

—Jenna Greditor, Editor, TWEENS & TEENS News

A recipe for success is presented with parents as role models and physical activities that are fun. Dr. Bartell's book contains hands-on instructions to guide parent and child in a non-stressful and at times, playful manner, using common sense and a dose of personal responsibility to gain a healthy lifestyle.

—Margaret M. Bores, P.T.A., M.S.Ed., Exercise Specialist

This book is a must read for parents wanting wholesome, balanced and practical tools for helping their children become healthier and lose weight when necessary. Dr. Susan supports you and your child all the way.

—**Sara Gragnolati,** Editor, *KIWI* magazine

Dr. Susan arrives just in time to offer wondrous emotional salvage for parents and children alike, along with brilliant eating pattern shifting that leads to a more healthful diet and weight loss. This book should be required reading for us all.

—**Stacy DeBroff,** best-selling author of *The Mom Book,* and founder, www.MomCentral.com

Dr. Susan untangles the world of why our kids overeat and how we as parents can help keep them healthy. Great bite-size pieces of info that are oh-so-yummy and easy to digest!

—**Pamela Atherton,** Host of award-winning radio show A Closer Look

Dr. Susan Bartell returns with another fantastic guide for both children and their parents. Though the book is geared towards the parent, its format and writing style make it engaging so that all ages will enjoy it and benefit. . . Use Dr. Susan's advice and start by changing the whole family's eating patterns. . . this book is a must-have for all parents!

—**Roundtable Reviews**

Inspirational and honest, a great resource for parents with overweight children, as well as parents who want to instill good eating habits within their families.

—**AnnMarie Evola,** Editor, *ParentGuide* (New York)

I work with many overweight kids struggling with the accompanying issues of low self-esteem, poor self-image and peer ridicule and rejection. Dr. Susan's wonderful, practical, parent-friendly guide just might put a significant crimp in my caseload! Bravo!

—**Dr. Vicki Panaccione,** Founder, Better Parenting Institute

Got kids? Then devour this book! Read this—if your family has food issues. Better yet, read this even if they don't. You'll feel a huge weight lifted off your shoulders and be totally prepared to keep your kids as healthy as can be.

—**Janene Mascarella,** Parenting & Family Life columnist, *The Long Island Exchange*

Dr. Susan has done it again! Her practical and useful guide assists parents in raising healthy kids by setting families up for success. She brings knowledge to a level of understanding that is necessary to make healthy lifestyle choices in everyday life.

—Jean Huelsing, RN, BSN, MEd, Founder, Camp Jump Start, CEO, Living Well Foundation

Once again Dr. Susan has presented an honest, thought-provoking and unflinching approach to the issues of weight loss and healthy lifestyle changes that puts parents on notice that these issues do not belong to our children alone, but are instead best handled as a family.

—Liza N. Burby, Editor, *Newsday's* Parents & Children magazine

A boon for families who are concerned about their children's eating habits and nutrition. Dr. Susan's real-world suggestions provide do-able models for beleaguered families. She educates adults so they can better educate and advocate for kids.

—Sandra Burt and Linda Perlis, Parents' Perspective, Inc., www.parentsperspective.org, Authors, *Raising a Successful Child* and *Washington, D.C. with Kids*

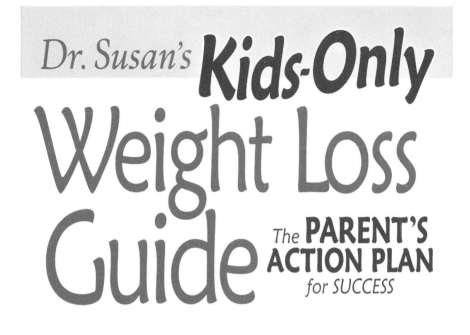

Dr. Susan's *Kids-Only*
Weight Loss Guide

The **PARENT'S ACTION PLAN** for *SUCCESS*

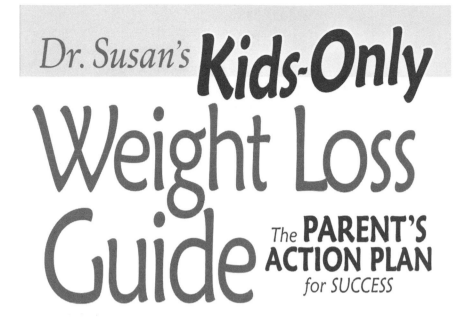

Dr. Susan's Kids-Only Weight Loss Guide

The PARENT'S ACTION PLAN for SUCCESS

DR. SUSAN S. BARTELL

Parent Positive Press
New York

Publisher's note: The information and advice in this book should not be used instead of medical advice. You should speak to your doctor about your health, especially about things that may need diagnosis or medical attention.

For bulk or special sales please call
(877) 885-BOOK (2665) or email info@parentpositive.com

Published by
Parent Positive Press
P.O. Box 118
Williston Park, NY 11596
http://www.girlsonlyweightloss.com/

ISBN-10: 0–9721502–1–8
ISBN-13: 978–0–9721502–1–7

First Printing

Cover design by George Foster
Interior design by Desktop Miracles

Publisher's Cataloging-in-Publication

Bartell, Susan S.
    Dr. Susan's kids-only weight loss guide : the parent's action plan for success / Susan S. Bartell.
        p. cm.
    Includes index.
    ISBN 0-9721502-1-8
    1. Obesity in children.   2. Weight loss.   3. Parent and child.   I. Title.   II. Title: Kids-only weight loss guide.
RJ399.C6B37   2007   618.92'398
                                                         QBI06-600411

For Max
Your birth made me a mother and with every day since,
your passion for life has taught me
how to be the best mother I can possibly be.
I love you.

For Lewis
You are my soul mate and ours is a true partnership.
I love you more than I can ever express in words alone.

For My Dad
Your love, support, and enthusiasm for my work means the world to me.
Thank you, I love you.

In Memory of Stuart
The most wonderful, warm loving father-in-law
I could have asked for.

Acknowledgments

I believe that it is impossible to write a book without enormous help and support from many people in a variety of capacities. It is my deepest pleasure to recognize and thank all those people who made it possible to realize my dream of having this book come to fruition.

First and foremost, I want to say a heartfelt thank you to my **Parents Advisory Group**. These remarkable people donated hours, weeks, and months of their time and life experience as well as giving an emotional commitment to enriching the lives of the parents reading the book. They gave of themselves through the usual hectic lives that we all lead, but sometimes even through extraordinary challenges of family illness and other unusual life stressors. They shared stories, suggested changes that improved and enriched each chapter, and through it all offered me such generous support and encouragement that I often wished they were sitting right in my office with me, rather than scattered all over the country! These truly wonderful individuals are: Peter Arango, Keith Benson, Maury Benson, Melinda DiCiro, Nicole Donoghue, Judy Jackson, David Larson, Gena Larson, Robyn Ratcliffe Manzini, Emily Roberts, Lois Scaglione, Jackie Schiff, Steven Schiff, and Ivy Woolf Turk. Thank you all from the bottom of my heart!

Several remarkable professionals helped to give this book greater depth and authority. Each gave generously of his or her knowledge and expertise, expecting nothing in return. I am truly grateful to these individuals for taking the time out of their already extremely busy lives to give to this project. They are: Sarita Dhuper, M.D., Judy Marshel, Ph.D., Rebecca Randall, M.S.W., Sarah Schmitt, M.A., Neville Golden, M.D., and Reed Mangels, Ph.D. Thank you all for helping to enrich my work and, even more, thank you for the important work that you do in the lives of parents and children.

I've had several other supporters along the way who have helped get this project off the ground and running, even as deadlines have loomed and almost passed! I want to tell each and every one of them how much I appreciate them for pitching in, staying up late and giving it their all! So I send out a huge thank you to George Foster, Sharon Castlen, Jacqui Brownstein, Susan Clark, Shawna Rocha, and Miranda Welsh. And although I have thanked Rebecca Randall, I would also like to thank *Common Sense Media* for generously providing me with Rebecca and with all the statistics in Chapter Three. I'd also like to thank Tagni McRae at the American Heart Association for her help in gathering information.

For me, every single book I write is, in some way, a family project and this one is no exception. My children are some of my greatest supporters and I am truly blessed to have their love and encouragement. As always, Max, Gillian, and Mollie, I love you to the stars, to the moon, to Brooklyn and back again!

I am very appreciative and grateful to have wonderful parents and an equally terrific mother-in-law, all of whom help me and facilitate my work in more ways than I can begin to say. Your incredible help (and bragging about me to your friends!) don't go unnoticed and I love you all.

As always, I owe my deepest gratitude to my husband, Lewis. It was only with his love, encouragement, help, and commitment to me and to our family that I was able to give this project the dedication that it deserved. Lew, you are my never-ending love.

SUSAN S. BARTELL, PSY.D.
January 2007

Table of Contents

Acknowledgments **7**

Introduction: Facing Your Child's Future:
                 Let's Make It Fabulous! **11**

One: "It's Just Baby Fat . . ." and Other Myths **15**

Two: Stepping onto the Road to Health **30**

Three: The Battle Begins Outside Your Front Door **40**

Four: Predictable Family Patterns **59**

Five: Feelings Might Make a Child Fat **86**

Six: The Real Road to a Healthier Child **108**

Seven: Yes, Your Child *Can* Eat Out Healthily **134**

Eight: Preventing and Understanding Eating Disorders
             (and Getting Help) **149**

Nine: Let's Get Moving (It's Easier Than You Think!) **156**

One Last Word . . . or Two **176**

Appendix One: Meet the Parents Advisory Group **179**

Appendix Two: Meet the Experts **186**

Appendix Three: Organizations, Websites, Books,
                    and Other Useful Information..........................**190**

Index **199**

Facing Your Child's Future: Let's Make It Fabulous!

Welcome! I'm so glad you're here. You have opened this book and started reading, which already tells me something important...you love your child and you're not sure where to turn for help. Well stop right here and take a deep breath because you're in the right place—I'm going to teach you the skills you need to help your child (whether a kindergartner or a fifth grader) feel and look better!

You've begun reading because you're struggling with a very real problem: *your child is overweight*. Perhaps the doctor (at the dreaded annual physical) told you or your child that s/he needs to lose weight, or maybe you've noticed it yourself when you compare your child to friends? Perhaps it crept up slowly or it could seem like it's happened all of a sudden.

You have probably noticed that in many painful ways your child is suffering for it—s/he may feel teased, left out, not very confident or even depressed, might not be able to keep up with others athletically, or you may witness sadness or meltdowns in clothing store fitting rooms or jealousy of siblings or friends who are not overweight. I'm sure it's painful for you too, even though you may have become quite good at hiding your feelings from your child.

Being overweight is hard for a child, I know because I became overweight as a teenager when I stopped figure skating and didn't replace it with any other form of exercise. I remember hating the feeling of not fitting into the fashionable clothes that I was desperate to wear, and thinking that the boy I liked wouldn't ever like a "fat girl." I also remember trying to diet, but then sneaking junk food up to my room after everyone had gone to sleep, because I didn't want my parents to see me eating it. It took me years to learn how to eat healthily, to take care of my body, to lose the weight, and to develop a good body image.

Now, as a parent of three children, I see the pressures that can interfere with good heath that my, and all kids, face in so many areas. There are pressures to fit into constantly changing and sometimes unrealistic fashions, unbelievable demands to resist the barrage of advertising for unhealthy food products, and the burden of ever-shrinking media stars making kids feel they might as well give up trying to be healthier. Of course, there are also the ever-present supersized portions of food everywhere we go. Our kids need our help to become healthier, not only physically, but emotionally as well.

Learning how to successfully help your overweight child is not as difficult to master as most people think, but it takes more than just good nutrition and exercise. I'm sure that none of the parenting books you've read, or those on how to raise a healthy child, has ever talked about the topics you'll learn about here.

- For one thing, you probably didn't know that there are seven Family Patterns that can lead to a child gaining too much weight. Take a look at Chapter Four and see which one fits your family.
- In Chapter Five I'll also show you how your child's—*and even your*—emotions can get in the way of your child's healthy eating and even cause your child to eat too much.
- It can be difficult to teach one's child how to eat healthily when we're not sure how to do so ourselves. But in Chapter Six, I'll give you all the tools you need to help your child eat healthfully. This will greatly improve his or her chances of becoming healthier and avoid weight gain.

- In addition, in Chapter Seven, I'll show you some special secrets for making sure that your child learns how to choose healthier, but still tasty foods, from the menu in a restaurant.
- It can be tough to get a child to exercise, but Chapter Nine has some fun and interesting ways to get your child moving so s/he won't even know it is exercise.

These are just a few of the special tools you'll learn. Now, we're almost ready to begin. But before we do, take a quick look through the Table of Contents because, aside from the highlights I've shared with you already, you will see many other important ideas—like how to help protect your child from developing an eating disorder (one of the greatest fears a parent has when trying to help a child to lose weight).

I've had some terrific and very smart experts help me write this book. You can learn more about them in Appendix Two. I've also had an incredible Parents Advisory Group—parents just like you, who read every chapter to make sure that the advice and information would really help you and your child. You can also read more about each parent in Appendix One. I thank each and every one from the bottom of my heart. Throughout the book, you'll also hear from other parents who have taken the time to share their thoughts and stories. They will remind you that you are not alone in your struggle.

Last, don't forget that in addition to being a psychologist who helps parents and kids, I'm also a mom with three children of my own. I know just how you feel and I'm with you all the way. So, I'd love to hear from you with comments, questions or ideas. You can reach me anytime at DrSusan@kidsonlyweightloss.com. Now, let's begin.

P.S.

I battled with how to represent both boys and girls equally throughout the book and decided that writing him/her and he/she on every page in every chapter would drive me, if not you crazy! I tried to be gender neutral whenever possible, and at other times . . . well, I did my best!

"It's Just Baby Fat"
...and Other Myths

ere's a bit of a conversation I heard between two moms talking to each other in the supermarket (I have to admit that I was eavesdropping in the fruit aisle!):

Mom #1: I'm shopping for healthy foods today—the doctor told me Melanie needs to watch **her** weight.

Mom #2: How can that be—she's only eight! Won't she just outgrow it? Isn't it just baby fat?

Mom #1: That's what I thought! But the doctor said that after about two years old it's not baby fat any more—it's just fat and it's not healthy!

Mom #2: Wow! I didn't know that, maybe I should take Freddy to see the doctor—I have a feeling I'll be here shopping for healthy foods too!

You may have also been surprised to find out that "baby fat" is not something kids naturally outgrow! Dr. Hilton Silver, a most wonderful pediatrician (and I must admit, my father!) told me that he must frequently explain to parents that it is far healthier for children to lose their "baby fat" as they leave toddlerhood than to keep it. In addition, he often needs to explain to parents that children won't lose this weight without eating more healthily and exercising.

In fact, the idea that children will naturally outgrow their "baby fat" is just one of the "medical myths" that parents believe about their children's weight and health. There are many others that parents think are true, but which unfortunately stand in the way of their children becoming truly healthy.

Medical Myths

We're going to start off with a quiz to test your Medical Myth knowledge. Answer each question True or False and then check your responses against the answer key. We'll devote the rest of the chapter discussing the Medical Myths. I'll give you the tools to recognize and correct these myths—by the time we reach the last page of the chapter you'll be amazed at how much more knowledge you'll already have about your child's health.

1. T F Given the opportunity, a child will always make the healthiest food choice available.

2. T F A chubby toddler will naturally slim down with age.

3. T F Children need limits when it comes to eating.

4. T F Your child will lose weight if you put her on the latest fad diet that worked for you.

5. T F Kids always lose weight as they go through puberty.

6. T F Genetics plays a part in a child's tendency to gain weight.

7. T F Kids don't need to exercise, they get enough in school.

8. T F The best way to have a healthy, slim child is to forbid all sugared, processed foods.

9. T F Much like an adult, all it takes is willpower for a child to lose weight.

10. T F It's best to monitor everything your child eats.

11. T F If the doctor hasn't told me my child is obese I don't have to worry.

12. T F If I tell my child she needs to eat more healthily, she'll develop an eating disorder.

Scoring: After checking out how you did on the quiz, don't forget to read Unmasking the Myths, to understand the answers.

1. False: Given the chance, kids won't always make the best choices.

2. False: A chubby toddler won't always slim down.

3. True: Children definitely need limits when it comes to food.

4. False: Fad diets are not a good choice for children.

5. False: Some children, especially girls, gain weight as they enter puberty.

6. True: Genetics is responsible for some, but not all, of a child's tendency to gain weight.

7. False: Children rarely get enough exercise as a part of their regular school day.

8. False: Denying your child any one type of food will encourage your child to want it even more.

9. False: Children need more than simply willpower to lose weight or be healthy.

10. False: Monitoring your child's eating will not aid weight loss and could be detrimental.

11. False: The word "obese" is a medical term that describes a certain percentage of being over a medically healthy weight. A child can be unhealthily overweight long before becoming medically obese.

12. False: Your child can't develop an eating disorder from conversation about beginning a healthy lifestyle.

Unmasking the Myths

So, how did you do? Each of the quiz questions represents a Medical Myth. Even if you scored well on the quiz, read the following section carefully because there is sure to be information that will help you jump-start your child on the road to better health.

MYTH #1:

Given the opportunity, a child will always make the healthiest food choice available

Even when children and teens are motivated to lose weight, they will *still* instinctively want to satisfy their taste buds before they think about their health. This is because they have not yet learned how to put their needs (health) before their desires. And, because in many cases, the most delicious choice will not be the healthiest, a child will often make the choice that is not best for her health. In fact, this continues to be a hard choice for many adults! In addition, children will not always consider the portion size of the foods that they choose, very often eating much larger portions than are healthy for them.

As a parent, it is your job to help your child meet this challenge in three ways:

1. By providing as many delicious tasting healthy alternatives as possible and by teaching your child that delicious can also be healthy (see Chapter Six for Sensational Substitutions).

2. By helping your child to make healthy choices when eating away from home (see Chapter Seven) so that she learns how to negotiate the available choices.

3. By working hard to live a healthy lifestyle yourself you can also model it for your child.

MYTH #2:

A chubby toddler will naturally slim down with age

Otherwise known as the "It's just baby fat" myth. As a parent, our natural instinct is to make sure that we are feeding our child enough. An infant can't tell us (except by crying) whether he is hungry. But a chubby baby assures us visually that we have not undernourished our little one. Without realizing it, we let the need for *visual* satisfaction that we have nourished our child, continue as our baby becomes a toddler and then a child. Before our eyes, the cherubic infant is now an overweight ten year old who *will not outgrow his baby fat no matter how much we wish he will*.

No matter how difficult it might be to admit it to yourself, it's time to banish this myth—whether your child is four or fourteen! Perhaps you need to take a look inside and ask yourself the following questions:

1. Does your child's "baby fat" make you feel like a better parent because it assures you that she's eating enough? You know now that this is a myth. Having an overweight child does not mean that you are a better parent. In fact, helping your child become healthier may make you an even better parent than you are already—you've already begun to help your child in a very meaningful way by reading this book!

2. Does the "baby fat" help you to feel that you can hold onto your "baby" for a bit longer, before she has to grow up and become a "big kid"? It is very hard to let our children grow up and separate from us, and that "baby fat" might give you the illusion that you're keeping her close. But, in reality, it's giving both you and your child a false sense of security. As your child grows up you can be close in different, just as wonderful ways, as when she was a baby. So, help her to let go of her baby fat and grow into a strong child or teenager. Take her hand and teach her how to do it.

3. Does calling it "baby fat" mean that you don't have to admit that it might be "real" fat? This can be the hardest question for many parents to answer. Be honest with yourself because your child's physical and emotional health is at the heart of your answer. It's okay to cry a few tears and it's okay to admit to having made some mistakes. There is no such thing as a perfect parent—not one of us is perfect, but we all keep trying.

MYTH #3:

Kids don't need to watch what they eat

It is a common myth that children should be allowed to eat whatever and whenever they want and that they will naturally regulate themselves to eat healthily. While this may be the case for a small number of children, it is the rare exception (which may be why you are reading *Kids-Only Weight Loss Guide*). Some parents think that because their child is not overweight it means he is self-regulating—not so. In fact, a child's weight is only one factor in his health. What's more, a slim child can very easily become an overweight teen or adult when healthy habits are not taught (and modeled) at a young age. In most cases an overweight child has not learned to self-regulate and therefore requires your help. The trick is how to help in a way that teaches your child to help himself, rather than making him dependent on you. Chapters Six and Seven will show you how to do this.

MYTH #4:

You and your child should go on diet together to lose weight

The best way to approach this myth is to say right up front that the word **diet** should not be included in a discussion about a healthy lifestyle for kids. There are two reasons for this:

Reason #1: No matter how overweight, a child needs to eat a variety of nutritious foods including those containing carbohydrates, proteins, and, YES, even fats! We will talk more about this in Chapter Six, but adult diets are not meant for children's growing bodies. These diets typically limit entire food groups (some aren't even healthy for adults). For example, high protein diets drastically limit carbohydrates and very low-fat diets rely far too much on carbohydrates and deprive children of healthy fats and protein that their bodies require for healthy body and brain development.

Reason #2: *A child's calorie requirements are not the same as those of an adult.* Most diets that an adult will follow in order to try and lose weight will be formulated around a certain number of calories a day—whether or not the diet tells you the actual number, or just tells you which foods to eat.

It is unlikely that this will be the correct number of calories for your child. It is very important that you speak to your child's doctor or to a pediatric nutritionist or dietician before making any drastic changes in your child's eating habits that are NOT specifically recommended for your child. Your child will be healthier and safer if you simply follow the guidelines of a professional and also the suggestions in this book.

MYTH #5:

Kids always lose weight as they go through puberty

Some parents of overweight kids eagerly await puberty because they hope that the otherwise hideous hormones of adolescence somehow have a silver lining that will miraculously transform their chubby child into a slim adolescent. And there are actually times when this does happen! But, not as often as one would hope and it also depends upon how overweight a child is to begin with, and also how quickly and how much they grow as they enter puberty. Here are two different illustrations of how puberty might affect a child:

Example #1: Kellie was quite chubby at 10 years old. She began puberty at eleven and between ten and fourteen she grew eight inches. By the time Kellie reached her full height of 5'4" at 15 years old, she had slimmed down considerably and could no longer be considered overweight.

Example #2: David was a very overweight 10 year old. He began puberty at eleven and although he grew a little taller each year he continued gaining weight through puberty and into his teens. By the time he had a real growth spurt at 15 years old, David was already extremely overweight and struggling to gain control of his body. His growth spurt was not enough to help him slim down and he was experiencing significant psychological damage from being overweight for so many years.

As you can see, puberty may or may not have a positive effect on your child's body and weight. What's more, as girls go through puberty their changing bodies typically gain some weight in order to accommodate widening hips and enlarging breasts. It can therefore be very difficult for an overweight preteen or teenage girl to lose weight without really making an effort.

If you have a tween or teen daughter struggling with her weight or body image, give her a wonderful gift, my other book: *Dr. Susan's Girls-Only Weight Loss Guide: The Easy, Fun Way to Look and Feel Good!* She'll really thank you for it and she can email me all her questions and comments right from the website www.girlsonlyweightloss.com.

For boys, weight loss during the early teen years can be challenging because a boy typically doesn't have a real growth spurt until later on. BUT, if you begin working with your tween or teen boy now to begin developing healthier habits then, WOW, when that growth spurt happens, he sure will thank you because he will see his body becoming strong and lean before his very own eyes! The knowledge you will gain in reading this book is a gift that you will give your children now and as they become teens and adults.

MYTH #6:

My child is overweight because of the bad genes he inherited, there's nothing I can do about it

Certainly, genetics does play a role in a child's tendency to be overweight. Body type, weight, heart disease, and cholesterol all run in families. But statistically, the rate of overweight children in the United States and in many other countries in the world has been increasing over the last twenty-five years, without *any* change in genetics! It's our environments that we've been steadily changing. You see, it's easier to blame genetics for many things that may actually be based in your family *environment* rather than your family genes. If you are overweight and so is everyone else in your family, you could say that it's because you all have an "overweight" gene. BUT, I'd argue that it's more likely because all the people in your family make eating and exercise choices that aren't particularly healthy. I think that by the time you finish this book, I will have helped you create a new gene—one for great knowledge, good decision making, and healthy kids and families. When you think you've got this gene, send me an email at DrSusan@kidsonlyweightloss.com.

MYTH #7:

Kids get enough exercise during the school day

The truth is that most children don't get enough exercise during the school day. Yes, they do attend physical education (PE) classes and they might have some time to run around on the playground during recess. But much of this time is spent in transit—to and from gym or the playground; not to mention classes that are canceled because of assemblies or playtimes that are rained out. In addition, lots of kids spend recess not moving their bodies at all, preferring rather to simply hang out chatting or playing with handheld video games.

Overweight children are particularly likely to choose this last option because they are often much more resistant to moving their body than those children who aren't overweight. As you might imagine, it's a bit of a vicious cycle—as an overweight kid, it can be physically difficult, tiring, and embarrassing to exercise your body, so you're reluctant to do so. Of course, exercising is exactly what your body needs to become healthier, but you avoid it and continue to gain (or at least not lose) weight!

To break this cycle children need outlets to exercise other than at school. In Chapter Nine, we will explore lots of really great, fun ways that you can help your child begin to get moving and you might even find that you're enjoying it too!

MYTH #8:

The best way to have a healthy, slim child is to forbid all sugar and processed foods

Take a minute and do this exercise.

1. Think of your favorite food.

2. Now, imagine that you have just been told that you can **never, ever** eat it again—**ever!!**

3. What's your first urge? To run out and get it and eat it, right? Of course, that's how we all feel when we're told we can't have something.

It's the very reason that diets almost always fail—because they're about depriving yourself of foods that you love in order to reduce the amount of food or calories you eat. But, it's extremely difficult to deprive yourself completely—whether you're an adult or a child—of foods that you love for more than a short period of time.

As an adult, you can end your own deprivation whenever you decide you've had enough, but as a child whose parent has decided to completely forbid candy, cookies or other supposedly "bad" foods, it's not as easy.

Think back to the experiment we just did. Most kids become obsessed with forbidden foods. At a friend's house they will eat as much junk food as possible—frequently overeating. But they won't tell mom or dad about it, choosing instead to harbor the guilty secret. They may also keep a secret stash in their room or school locker. They live with the constant internal battle to find moderation. In fact, this is one of parents' greatest fears: If I talk to my child about her weight, she will get an eating disorder! In Chapter Eight I will teach you everything you need to know to help your child lose weight and become healthier without needing to worry that she will develop an eating disorder

Just as it is confusing to have a home filled with junk food and no rules around about when to eat it, it is also stressful to have no junk food at all. A child needs to know that there is no "forbidden fruit" and she also needs to learn how to consume all foods in moderation—**this is arguably THE most important skill that an overweight child must learn**. In Chapter Six, we will discuss this in great detail because I will show you how to teach your child about portion control, about how to learn to pay attention to one's body, and how to learn not to binge or eat secretly so you can raise a healthy child who is not at risk for developing an eating disorder.

MYTH #9:

Much like an adult, all it takes is willpower for a child to lose weight

Here's the list of the things that a child needs, in order of importance, in order to lose weight:

1. A supportive family (that really lives the life they are teaching)

2. Knowledge and information

3. The right foods and the chance to exercise

4. Willpower (which is actually that the desire to be healthy becomes greater than the need to give in to the immediate, short-term pleasure of eating)

Willpower is last on the list because it truly is the least important! A child cannot make a big, long-lasting life change, such as losing weight, without enormous support and help from a parent or other family members.

It is therefore **very** important to make sure that your child feels that this is a team effort—something that you are doing together. Throughout *Kid's-Only Weight Loss Guide* we will discuss many ways that you will be able to help your child become successful weight losers, thereby becoming winners!

MYTH #10

It is best to monitor everything your child eats

Parents sometimes believe that watching and regulating everything your child eats will ensure that she loses weight, since you will be controlling it. Actually this can backfire on you **very badly** for two reasons:

1. Your child won't learn to make good choices for himself, which means that when he goes off to high school or college he won't have learned the skills he needs to make sure he stays healthy without you being there to help him.

2. If you monitor everything your child eats it can be incredibly stressful for your child, causing arguments, secretive eating, and lots of guilt. We will delve into this in great detail when we get to Chapter Four. But if this is a big concern for you, as it is for lots of parents, feel free to jump there right now! Just don't forget to come back.

MYTH #11:

If the doctor hasn't told me my child is obese I don't have to worry

Obesity is a medical term and a person (adult or child) is considered obese when his or her body mass index (BMI—a number calculated using a person's height and weight) is above a medically acceptable range for that person's age. When your BMI is too high it means that your weight is too high for your height. So, if your doctor has told you that your child's weight or BMI are in the obese range, you certainly should worry.

It is important to note that BMI does not take into account lean muscle mass, which means that if your child happens to be particularly muscular he may have a high BMI, as an overweight child would. Most doctors will observe a child's body and be able to tell the difference between a muscular child and one that is overweight. But if your doctor is strict about utilizing BMI to determine whether a child is overweight and you don't agree because you recognize that your child's body is composed of muscle rather than fat (due to being an athlete, for example), it is your duty to speak up to the doctor—and perhaps find a new doctor.

But, if the doctor hasn't told you that your child is obese, it doesn't necessarily mean your child is healthy! This is because your child can be overweight—significantly overweight—without being statistically obese. So, if you have any questions about your child's health, don't focus too much on the terminology being used. Instead, as you read the rest of this guide think about the skills you are learning to help your child to feel and look healthier and more confident, no matter what the label!

MYTH #12:

If I tell my child she needs to eat more healthily, she'll develop an eating disorder

In this culture where the media bombards us with super-skinny models and size 00 clothes, it is understandable for a parent to worry that any suggestion that a child is overweight could trigger an overweight child to become overly concerned with being thin. Since not only girls, but increasingly boys too, are at risk for developing eating disorders, this can be a concern for the parents of both genders if an overweight child becomes overly concerned with losing weight.

But, it is important to recognize that supportive, helpful, noncritical, nonjudgmental conversations that focus on weight loss to improve health will not trigger a child to develop an eating disorder. Children become at risk for self-critical feelings and behaviors when they believe they are failing themselves or their parent in the process of losing weight. It is therefore extremely important to choose your words with great care so that they reflect sensitivity to your child's feelings about her weight and body image.

Throughout the book we will talk about the best words to use to talk to your child about his or her weight to ensure a positive body image and healthy weight loss without risking the possibility of an eating disorder. In Chapter Eight, I will share some of the early warning signs of eating disorders so you know what to look for and can seek help if necessary.

❧ ❧ ❧ ❧ ❧

Now you know the myths, you're ready for some facts! Let's begin by figuring out for sure whether your child really is overweight. Then we'll tackle the really tough job of how to first approach your child about beginning to make the necessary changes toward becoming healthier. Even if you've already taken some of these steps, you'll definitely learn some new facts and skills so don't skip the next chapter . . .

Stepping onto the Road to Health

Facing the Physical Facts

When Margaret first brought her son Sean (9) to see me she thought he had poor social skills. I met with Sean several times, as well as with Margaret and also spoke with Sean's teacher. After the evaluation, at a follow-up meeting, Margaret was shocked and a little angry when I suggested that perhaps Sean's weight was interfering with his self confidence. "He's just a big kid!," she told me. Over time, which included a meeting with the pediatrician and further conversations with Sean and Margaret, Margaret came to understand that Sean would not only be healthier, but would feel better if he could lose some weight. Sean's doctor also explained to Margaret that being "a big kid" wasn't healthy for Sean—physically or emotionally.

Often you just know that your child is overweight—it's obvious from looking at your child, from trying to buy clothes, or from comparisons with other children. But sometimes (like for Margaret), despite what the doctor says, it can be really hard to *admit* to yourself that your child needs to lose or stop gaining weight.

In fact, this is often the most difficult part because acknowledging it can make you feel like you have somehow failed your child by not being able to keep him or her healthier. Tania, the mother of Shantal (10) shared this exact feeling with me:

" For two years the doctor has been saying that Shantal needs to lose weight. To be honest, I kept telling myself that she wasn't that fat, that she eats okay, and that the doctor is overreacting. But, last week I saw her in a dance recital and I nearly cried. It was so obvious that she needed to lose weight! I think that the whole time I was trying to convince myself that she wasn't overweight was because I didn't want to admit that I, as a mother, had messed up. It was a shock for me to admit it, even to myself. But now, at least I'm ready to do the work to help her become healthier. "

Since most parents feel at least a little bit like Tania, here's a chance to help yourself really come to terms with whether your child needs to lose weight. Take the quiz below, then calculate your score and read your results. You don't have to share your results with anyone—except maybe your child's doctor. We will talk more in Chapter Five about how to help you overcome your feelings of guilt and all the other emotions connected to having an overweight child. For now, we'll focus on helping you to take the first steps to identify your child's needs and help him or her to become healthier.

Answer as honestly as you can, choosing the response that is closest to accurate for your child and family.

1. Compared to other children around the same age and height, my child is
   a. about the same body size.
   b. a little heavier/bigger.
   c. a lot heavier/fatter.

2. At dinnertime my child eats
   a. one average helping of food and sometimes a second of the same size.
   b. at least two large helpings and sometimes more.
   c. not very much, she's usually not hungry because she snacks a lot during the day.

3. Clothes shopping for my child
   a. is really difficult—the size that fits around his waist is usually much too long. Elasticized waists are the best.
   b. isn't a big deal, she seems to fit easily into most clothing in most stores.
   c. used to be easier, but now seems to be more of a challenge because it's harder to find things that fit.

4. My child's favorite type of exercise is
   a. the fast moving, nonstop kind that makes you sweat a lot and your heart beat fast.
   b. moderate activity that increases your heartbeat a little and makes you sweat a bit—with frequent breaks.
   c. raising his arm to click the TV remote or move the computer mouse.

5. The amount of exercise my child gets is
   a. daily (at least 6 hours a week).
   b. three to four times a week (at least three hours a week).
   c. less than three hours a week.

6. Most of my child's favorite foods are in which group?

    a.   pasta, rice, bread, crackers

    b.   meat, poultry, fruit, vegetables, cheese, peanut butter, pizza

    c.   chicken nuggets, burgers, hot dogs, fries

7. My child eats

    a.   for the most part only when she is hungry.

    b.   when meals and snacks are served.

    c.   when bored or any time food is not restricted.

8. Compared to the rest of the family my child is

    a.   heavier than most of us.

    b.   about the same—we're all at a healthy weight.

    c.   about the same—we're all a little overweight.

9. The last time my child went for a check-up, the doctor

    a.   told me he needs to lose a little weight (or at least not gain weight as he grows and stretches out).

    b.   said she is in good health or didn't say anything at all.

    c.   said that he is overweight and needs to begin an immediate weight loss plan.

10. When my child walks or runs she

    a.   might get a little out of breath, but can do it without too much trouble.

    b.   hardly ever makes it to the endpoint with gasping for breath or stopping.

    c.   gets out of breath but can finish if pushed hard.

11. The total amount of sugar sweetened soda (pop), sports drinks, iced tea, lemonade and orange, apple, and other juices that my child drinks is approximately

    a.   one cup (8 oz) a day or less.

    b.   between one and three cups a day.

    c.   more than three cups a day.

12. The amount of water, seltzer, or club soda that my child drinks is approximately

    a. one cup (8 oz) a day or less.

    b. between one and three cups a day.

    c. more than three cups a day.

Scoring:

1.	a = 3	b = 2	c = 1
2.	a = 3	b = 1	c = 2
3.	a = 1	b = 3	c = 2
4.	a = 3	b = 2	c = 1
5.	a = 3	b = 2	c = 1
6.	a = 1	b = 3	c = 2
7.	a = 3	b = 2	c = 1
8.	a = 1	b = 3	c = 2
9.	a = 2	b = 3	c = 1
10.	a = 3	b = 1	c = 2
11.	a = 3	b = 2	c = 1
12.	a = 1	b = 2	c = 3

32-36: Healthy and Happy. Congratulations Your child is eating and exercising in the healthiest way possible and has the healthy body to show it. What's more, it sounds like your whole family is making some really healthy decisions. You should be proud of yourself! Use the rest of the book to learn the nutritional and exercise facts that you didn't know, get some new ideas to jump start your routine, and brush up on your healthy eating out strategies.

20-31: Chubby Ready for Change. Your child is probably showing signs of struggling with an overweight body, but you may not have wanted to acknowledge it before now. This is an excellent time to be reading this book and beginning to make the changes necessary to helping your child become healthier. The longer you wait to start, the harder it is to help your child—his self-esteem may already be suffering and peer pressure can make it tough as your child moves into older grades. Your doctor may not yet be raising the medical red flag. But as a parent you're probably seeing the signs of clothing that is a bit too tight, or unhealthy eating choices. Being proactive is important. You can feel good that you're ready to take the steps necessary to help your child feel better about her body before it becomes much more difficult.

12-19: Suffering in Solitude. Your child is undoubtedly really struggling with his weight. For many children being overweight, not knowing how to lose weight and then giving up and eating more, are a vicious cycle that keep kids trapped for years, into adulthood. It can impact deeply on self-esteem, on a child's social life, and on many other aspects of a child's sense of well being. It is of the utmost importance that you take all the steps throughout this guide to help your child begin to look and feel healthier. I will be here with you every step of the way.

The Medical Must

Of course, you can't rely on a quiz to tell you for a medical certainty whether your child needs to lose weight, or exactly how much. For that, it's really important that you take your child to see his or her pediatrician—after all, your child's physical and emotional health are both at stake!

It is very important to have your child's doctor check your child's height **and** weight—not just weight! You can't tell if a child is overweight simply by what the scale says. If your child is tall, he or she will weigh more but will not be overweight. For example, if your son's weight is in the 50th percentile and so is his height—he is well proportioned. On the other hand, if your daughter's height is in the 50th percentile and her weight is in the 90th, then she is overweight.

I spoke with Dr. Sarita Dhuper, a really wonderful pediatrician who specializes in helping kids lose weight and lead healthier lives. Dr. Dhuper explained that the most accurate method we use for assessing whether a child is overweight is to calculate her body mass index (BMI), which is calculated by looking at a child's height and weight and then comparing these on a standard graph for children of the same age.

If your child's BMI falls below the 85th percentile for BMI (meaning that only 85 percent of children have a BMI the same or higher) it means your child's weight is healthy for his height. If the BMI is above the 85th percentile and less than the 95th percentile your child is considered to be at risk for becoming overweight, and if the BMI is more than the 95th percentile your child is already overweight. Also, if there is a rapid jump in BMI from year to year it's a warning sign to begin a healthy eating and exercise plan right away to reduce this rapid weight gain before your child's BMI reaches the 95th percentile.

So, remember when it comes to a child's weight:

The number on the scale means nothing when looked at alone.
It is only important relative to height.

Although this next idea may seem obvious, I've worked with many parents of tall children who are upset about their child's weight simply because the number on the scale seems high. So, remember to resist the urge to focus on the scale, and instead, focus on your child as a *whole person*. Even your child's stage of development is a part of the picture. In fact, this is a message your will hear from me often. Your child is a complex, many-sided person and we will make sure to recognize all of these parts as we go through this book. After your child is weighed and measured, ask the doctor to explain the numbers and make a recommendation to you about whether your child would benefit from losing weight or perhaps trying to stretch out.

The Stre-e-e-e-tch

In many cases the doctor will tell you that your child doesn't need to lose weight, as long as he doesn't gain much weight as he grows over the next year or two. This will cause your child to "stretch out" as he gets taller. When children stretch out like this the result is **exactly the same as** when they actually lose weight. Therefore, everything we discuss in this book applies in absolutely the same way for parents who are hoping to maintain their child's weight through a growth period as for parents who have been told by the doctor that their child should actually lose weight.

Hide the Home Scale

After you have learned the pediatrician's recommendation for weight loss you may have the urge to reweigh your child at home or to weigh her periodically as you begin to help her lose weight. *Resist the urge!* **Don't weigh your child at home!**

Checking your child's weight can cause her to become self-conscious and preoccupied with the numbers on the scale. This can be the precursor to her becoming at risk for developing an eating disorder—this can be true for boys and girls (more in Chapter Eight). In addition, if the numbers on the scale don't go down as your child hopes or expects she may begin to feel that she's failing you and herself. If they don't go down the way you hope, *you* may begin to feel that she's failing you—clearly, none of these is healthy for your relationship with your child or for your child's emotional health.

Instead, concentrate on making healthier choices for your child and confine the weighing and measuring to the doctor's office as often as the doctor recommends. If your child feels more comfortable being weighed in the room alone with the doctor, it is fine, even advisable, to respect this wish. You should protect your child's pride by discussing the findings with the doctor at another time when your child is not in the room.

Let the Doctor Do the Dirty Work

When the numbers on the scale and charts confirm that your child is overweight, the most difficult next step is how to talk to your child about it. In fact, in most cases it should be the doctor that speaks to your child about his or her weight.

BUT, I suggest that you speak privately with the doctor prior to the scheduled meeting between your child and the doctor, simply to ensure that the meeting between them will be a positive experience for your child. The conversation should include the following:

1. Thank the doctor for meeting with your child and then say that you'd like to preface the rest of the conversation by saying that you hope you're not being presumptuous by making a couple of suggestions that you think will help your child.

2. Next, explain that you the want the meeting to be a **very** positive experience for your child and that you don't want your child to feel that the doctor is being critical.

3. Suggest that the doctor talk about focusing on becoming healthier rather than thinner and tell the doctor that you, the parent, are making a commitment to beginning to have a healthier home for your child.

4. Thank the doctor again and then be open to any comments/ discussion the doctor may have.

After the Meeting

The most important moment is not when the doctor speaks to your child, but right afterwards. The doctor has brought your child to a crossroad and offered your child a chance to step onto the long road to good health. You have the chance to support this first step or, alternatively, you can allow your child to continue on the easy, well-trodden path he (and perhaps your entire family) is already taking—the road of being overweight.

Of course, this crossroad doesn't always happen at the doctor's office. Some kids come to the realization that they need to lose weight without any help from the doctor after being teased in school one too many times, after taking a health class, or following a particularly demoralizing clothes shopping experience. Sometimes you reach the crossroad before your child does. Perhaps that's the reason you are reading this book. But it doesn't really matter—when they come to that crossroad, the question remains—are you going to support your child on the journey to better health?

Sandi was faced with just this question when her daughter Megan left the doctor's office in tears.

"I hate Dr. Lynn!" said Megan, "She's the worst doctor ever—she told me that I need to be healthier and exercise some more! I bet she thinks I'm fat!" Sandi was heartbroken to see Megan so upset, and it took all her willpower not to wrap her arms around Megan and tell her she was right about Dr. Lynn.

"Megan, sweetie, you know, I think Dr. Lynn is right—actually I think our whole family all needs to get healthier and exercise more. We'll start to work on it together—today!"

❧ ❧ ❧ ❧ ❧

So, what about you—is your child at the crossroad? Are you? I offer you the choice, right here, right now. Choose health for your child it is perhaps the most important gift you can give your child, one that will last an entire lifetime and one that could very well lengthen that lifetime. Take your child's hand and step onto the road. I'm with you. Let's go.

The Battle Begins Outside Your front Door

One important step down the road to your child's weight loss and better health is to become aware that each day you and your child will be confronted by potentially negative forces from the outside world that can interfere with even your best efforts to help your child look and feel better. Remember Darth Vader from *Star Wars?* Well, the negative forces are something like that! But once you and your child learn what they are and can recognize them when you see them, then suddenly their power over you quickly diminishes and even vanishes!

So, by the end of this chapter you will have the confidence to **recognize** and **combat** the potentially undermining effects of eight Negative Force Factors. Then you will be well on your way to being not only more educated, but healthier too! By the way, if you think I've missed any Negative Force Factors, feel free to email and tell me at DrSusan@kidsonlyweightloss.com.

Negative Force Factor #1:

Ads That Overwhelm

Did you know that kids see one food commercial for every *five* minutes of TV on Saturday mornings and that over 80 percent of foods advertised during TV shows targeted at kids are for fast food, snack food, and sweets! Amazing isn't it? I didn't know this either until I spoke to Rebecca Randall at *Common Sense Media*, which is a nonprofit organization dedicated to helping parents gain the knowledge and information necessary to make the best media decisions for their children (you can find out more about *Common Sense Media* and Rebecca in the Appendices).

All this advertising has an enormous impact on children, causing them to want to eat what they see advertised—whether it is healthy or not. So, in many cases, when your child asks, then begs, then begs some more, then wears you down and you purchase the food that is new, cool, "in" or an otherwise "must have," it's because your child has seen it on TV—or in another child's lunchbox (who saw it on TV).

The power of TV advertising is so strong that it's not only children, but also parents who become convinced to purchase food products that may not be the healthiest for their child. The advertisers count on the idea that if you watch an advertisement enough times, you'll eventually become convinced to buy their product. And the more often you and your children see advertising messages, the more ingrained they become in your mind. TV advertising is *that powerful!*

> **Try this experiment.** The next one-hour block of weekend time that your child watches TV, together with your child, count how many ads your see for food, drinks or snacks. Note how many of these are targeted directly to children. Now, multiply this by the number of hours your child watches TV a week. The results will astound you and make for a great conversation with your child. The numbers for my three kids were seven, ten, and nine—what were yours?

Another way that TV food advertising affects kids, is that it makes them want to eat and drink while they're watching TV.

So, when the ad for soda comes on, your child might jump up and grab a can from the fridge, or when the ad for cookies comes on, he dips into the bag of cookies. Think back to the experiment we just did—how many times might that be happening in your house in a day? A week? A month? In fact, research shows that for each hour of TV kids watch, they eat an average of 167 more calories than kids who don't watch TV. What's more, a preschooler's risk of obesity jumps 6 percent for every hour of TV watched and it *leaps 31 percent if the TV is in their bedroom.*

You may be interested to note that adults are also suggestible when it comes to what they see on the small screen—remember digging for that pint of ice cream in the freezer you'd all but forgotten the last time you saw a seductive ice cream ad on TV! It's important to be aware of this as you're trying to help your child.

These are serious and scary statistics. While I'm not suggesting that you throw the TV out the window (well, maybe . . .), we do need to consider how to make changes that will impact on TV viewing. So, now that you understand the Negative Force Factor, its time to fight back!

LAUNCH YOUR ATTACK

1. **Control TV viewing.** Clearly, the less TV your child watches the better. But, mainly, it's the *advertising time you're trying to limit.* So you are best to stick with noncommercial TV whenever possible (often easier with younger children). Then as much as is practical, prerecord your children's shows or record/DVR them and zoom through commercials. You may not be able to do it all the time, but do it as much as you can!

2. **Be clear with your children that you will not purchase foods simply because they are advertised on TV.** Instead, using this book to help you, begin developing guidelines for the types of foods that you will consider purchasing. Teach your children these guidelines (you may want to jump to Chapter Six for how to begin to do this). Soon, your children will become so familiar with the rules, they'll stop asking!

3. **No endless snacking while watching TV.** One healthy and *limited* snack—no refills...it doesn't matter what ads come on during the breaks. And that goes for you too while you're watching with your child.

4. **Educate your children.** Teach them that TV advertising is designed to make food seem more attractive. Explain that nutritional information is deliberately left out and that ads are strategically placed depending on the viewing audience. Teach them that advertisers profit financially from you purchasing their products, and that you—mom or dad—care about your child's health, but that not all food companies care in the same way. The more knowledge your child has the less power the advertising will have.

Negative Force Factor #2:

Food Is the Star of the Show

For some time now, we've been seeing a steady increase in product placements in both movies and TV shows. Product placement is when a product company pays a movie or TV show producer to have their product placed in the hands of an actor.

For example, if an actor in a movie is seen drinking Coca-Cola, rather than a no-name brand or a Pepsi, it's probably because Coke paid the movie producer to have the Coke placed in that actor's hand, hoping that everyone watching the movie would be more likely to buy a Coke next time they were shopping for soda. It's simply another form of advertising, and much like blatant TV ads, it has a significant effect on kids. It not only sways them to want that product, but to also want a soda right then (remember Negative Force Factor #1).

But, in some ways, product placement has an even more powerful effect on kids (and arguably adults too) than regular advertising because they associate the product with the actors they adore. What's even more seductive is that most of these stars are extremely thin girls and thin, muscular guys—all that an overweight child or teen desperately wishes he or she could look like. Notably, advertising that uses paid celebrities has a similar impact on kids and teens.

If the star wasn't drinking or eating a name brand product, there would be no need for the scene, no need for the association and no need for the struggling overweight child to feel a deep internal conflict, that as a parent it's important for you to understand.

In a conversation I had with Kevin (11) he expressed it more eloquently than I ever could:

> **"** Dr. Susan, I know I'm overweight, and I'm trying really hard to get healthier, but how come all the guys on TV get to eat everything that they want and they never gain weight—it's really frustrating! **"**

Product placement affects younger children as well, arguably, in an even more overwhelming way. When their favorite character or cartoon is placed *onto* the snack, candy or fast food—as a way to market and sell that product to young children—it becomes, for most children, almost impossible to resist. In fact, almost every major children's TV program has a licensed line of merchandise that is used to sell products, including sugary cereals and other food and drinks high in fat and calories.

What's more, Rebecca informed me that the food and beverage industry spends $10 billion (yes, that's a B) a year marketing to children and teens and that marketers reach out to kids beginning nearly from birth so that they develop brand loyalty! So that when promotional tie-ins to movies and TV shows land squarely in every child friendly fast food meal, it is up to you to recognize the powerful pull of the media, as exploited by the food companies and fight against it for the health of your child.

LAUNCH YOUR ATTACK

1. Educate your child! The next time you're in the movies and you see an actor eating or drinking a name-brand product lean over and whisper "Wow, look at that, I bet [*name brand*] paid the movie producer a lot to have their soda/pizza/candy in this movie. Pretty smart way of advertising huh!" Then after the movie, recall the moment and explain to your child about how this is really advertising. Your child will think it's really cool that they now know what's going on and they'll be on the look out for it, each time you go to the movies.

Don't be afraid to talk to young children about product placement and promotional tie-ins. As a fun experiment purchase the exact same product—one with a tie-in and one without (cereal is a good example of this). Do a "blind taste test" with your child to demonstrate that the food tastes exactly the same, regardless of what or who is on the box. Children as young as five or six can begin to grasp this concept and it's important to begin teaching it this young.

2. **In line with number 1, resist the urge to purchase products simply because they are associated with TV (or other) characters that your child likes.** In fact, this is a reason **not** to buy them! Your child may not be happy in the moment, but if you are consistent in your refusal to bend to this type of blatant marketing, not only will your child get used to it, but he will eventually become a more educated shopper too. Of course your child's *health* will also benefit from the reduction in junk food and fast food.

Negative Force Factor #3:

The Internet and the Cell Phone

The Internet is fast becoming the new way that advertisers are reaching out and grabbing the attention of children. They are doing so in some stealthy ways about which you, as a parent, may not even be aware.

Advergaming is a fairly recent phenomenon in which online or video games are embedded with a brand's message to promote the use of one or more of that brand's products. In a groundbreaking study (2006), the Kaiser Family Foundation selected nearly 100 companies that advertise on TV heavily during children's programming. They found that of these companies, fully 85 percent of them also had corporate or brand websites specifically for children under 12 years old. These websites are created to look like fun, lively, nonthreatening, and safe play places, but are really advergames, specifically designed to promote the brand and the products.

It is of great importance to note that in *many* cases children do not even realize that they are on a website that is advertising a product. They think they are playing a fun game and **have no idea that this game is actually just an advertisement!** But even more important, in even *more instances* I have found that many parents **do not know** that their children are on advergaming sites and that they are being inundated, practically brainwashed, with advertising through the games they are playing. Without looking closely, it is sometimes hard to tell that the innocent looking game a child is playing is actually an ad for sweetened cereal, soda, ice cream, candy or cookies.

Food companies reach older children through technology as well. As I learned from *Common Sense Media*, when preteens and teens buy candy and chips, their purchase may come with an offer of free music downloads, ring tones or wallpaper for their cell phones. Of course, they're routed to a website, which includes more advertising. In addition, once the food company has their phone number or email address (in order to send them the free downloads) the kids are inundated with even more advertising disguised as games, contests, and activities. Did you know about this? I didn't. As parents, we owe it to our children to become aware, educated and then to teach them!

LAUNCH YOUR ATTACK

1. **Keep your computer centrally located so you can keep an eye on what sites your children are viewing and using—it's a good habit to start while your child is young.** While advergaming can be harmful, it certainly doesn't have the potential for danger that many of the Internet experiences older children encounter. If your children get used to having the computer in a public area rather than in their bedroom, you will have less to worry about later on. If you feel that you'd really like your child to have a computer in the bedroom to be able to do schoolwork or play games, refrain from installing Internet capability.

2. **Sit with your children while they're online and inquire as to the sites they're using.** If you see them on an

advergaming site, you don't necessarily need to forbid it, but be sure to educate them as you did with Negative Force Factor #2. Explain how this is really advertising in disguise and how the product keeps showing up throughout the game. Tell them that it's "tricky advertising" but now they won't be fooled anymore. Suggest that they keep their eyes open for it on other sites and let you know if they see it anywhere else. They'll be proud to show you how smart they are!

3. **Be aware of how your older child is using a cell phone.** Educate your child about how food companies use technology to advertise to youth. Tell your child that they are not allowed to give their cell phone number to strangers, including for advertising purposes, not matter how cool the offer. Since you are paying for the phone, you are allowed to make this request—you can take the phone away if your child does not comply! This is your right as a parent.

Negative Force Factor #4:

Even School Isn't Safe from the Food Fight (and I Don't Mean in the Cafeteria)

The food and beverage industry knows that the best place to reach kids is where they spend most of their time—at school. And unfortunately in many cases, schools choose not to sufficiently protect students from product marketing and advertising that creeps into students' school days in many different ways. For example, vending machines are in practically every high school and as well as many middle and elementary schools. Many of these vending machines are sponsored by food and beverage companies.

Vending machines, whether or not they are sponsored, are typically filled with junk food (because that's what kids buy). Despite the recent law banning the sale of soft drinks in elementary schools, other sugary drinks, along with the chocolate bars, cookies, and chips are still available to students. Schools receive significant revenues from these machines and are therefore reluctant to take them out, or even turn them off during lunch hours—despite this being a compromise frequently suggested by parents and other watchdogs of children's health. Similar snacks are also available at student stores and snack bars.

But these are just the start. Beginning in elementary school, powerful food marketing toward students has already begun in full force in many other ways. Big business believes that money is well spent on advertising and marketing to kids because not only do they have a powerful influence on parents' spending, but they also develop brand loyalty beginning very young—long before they have the ability to actually spend money.

For this reason billions of marketing and advertising dollars in schools are spent in many different ways to reach and influence the eating behavior of children. For example, food companies sponsor contests (like read-a-thons and box-top collections) and schools receive products. Food companies also spend enormous amounts of advertising and promotional dollars on direct advertising, underwriting the costs of scoreboards, banners and even sponsoring textbooks. You may even see ads in school gyms, cafeterias, food carts, and locker rooms.

In about 30 percent of middle and high schools in the United States about seven million teens in about 11,000 schools are exposed to direct advertising through Channel One, a for-profit, classroom TV channel that shows twelve minutes of teen-directed news a day, including two minutes of commercials. Channel One regularly shows ads for candy, fast food, chips, and sodas to a captive, easily influenced audience who surely believe that if they're seeing it in school, it can't be bad!

For the most part parents are unaware of the steady onslaught of sometimes subtle, sometimes in-your-face advertising and marketing of nonnutritional food products that children are faced with in school on a regular basis.

LAUNCH YOUR ATTACK

1. **Once again, it's about opening your child's eyes to the role that advertising plays in the world and particularly at school.** When food advertising or marketing takes place on school grounds under different forms, take the time to teach your child about it and why it is important not to simply accept it at face value. The more you teach, the more your child will learn not to just accept that everything they are exposed to at school is in their best interest. This is an unfortunate, but important fact of life.

2. **Beginning at a very young age, do not allow your child to spend her money freely on food.** When you give an allowance, it is okay to say that it is not to be spent on junk food—including vending machines or snack bars at school. Make clear rules about what "lunch money" can be spent on and have consequences for these rules being broken. Remember, you are the parent, it is your money and you are allowed to make rules and enforce them!

3. **Speak up to the administration at your children's school.** If enough parents complain, perhaps *your* school will do the right thing and begin to make your child's school a healthier place for your child and future generations of students. There are resources online and in Appendix Three of this book that can help you become even further educated so that you can continue to advocate for your child's health.

Negative Force Factor #5:

Airbrushed Magazine Models, Itsy-Bitsy Actresses and Perfect Bodied Guys

My 10-year-old daughter shook her head with exasperation recently as she looked at the cover of a women's magazine.

"Mommy, why do the models on these magazines look so perfect? Don't they know that it makes the rest of us feel bad about ourselves?" I think she voiced the feelings of just about every child, overweight or not— and not just girls! In fact, the number of men's magazines are increasing with perfectly-muscled young men on every cover.

Being surrounded by seemingly perfect models, anorexic starlets, and famous guys with six-pack abs and small waists and can make an overweight child feel like giving up, or not even trying to lose weight. It can all seem so hopeless! What's more, reality becomes distorted—is this how you're supposed to strive to look? Sometimes even parents forget that this shouldn't be our goal for our child.

The reality is that in many cases the media icons that kids (and sometimes adults) worship are at an unhealthily low weight and the magazine models are airbrushed. We need to remember this so that we don't put too much pressure on our kids to be too thin and so they don't put too much pressure on themselves. It is this kind of pressure that can lead to an eating disorder (see Chapter Eight).

LAUNCH YOUR ATTACK

1. **Limit the number of fashion (men's and women's) and entertainment (the ones that update you about the lives of the stars) magazines you have in your home.** If they have particularly offensive covers, tear them off and throw them away. It may make them a bit harder for you

> to identify, but **much** better for your child's body image and self-esteem.
>
> **2.** Limit the amount of "life of the stars" TV you let your children watch.
>
> **3.** Resist the urge to comment positively about a super-thin actor or actress's body in front of your child. If your child makes a positive comment about someone extremely thin, respond by saying, "it's good to be healthy, but being too thin isn't good for your body either."

Negative Force Factor #6:

Poisonous Peers

Life in the classroom, on the ball field, on the playground, and just about everywhere else can be very tough for an overweight child and he may not even tell you about it. Children are often ashamed to tell their parents that they have been teased about their weight and instead they keep it inside, becoming sad, angry, withdrawn, lethargic or even depressed.

Since depression in children doesn't always look like classic adult depression, you may not even know that your child isn't happy. Instead you may see a child that is distracted, silly, moody, having a hard time with schoolwork or homework, or unwilling to spend time with peers. Your child might want to sleep a lot, or have trouble sleeping and you may see signs of anger, moodiness or changes in personality.

If you see changes in your child's behavior, or if you suspect, have heard, or if your child has told you he or she has been teased about being overweight *this is not something to ignore—even if your child asks you to do so.* Your child needs your help, your advocacy. There are different ways to handle it depending on your child's age.

LAUNCH YOUR ATTACK

1. **If your child is in elementary school, call the teacher and, if necessary, the school counselor or principal to let them know what happened.** This is a form of bullying and it needs to be stopped immediately. Your expectation should be that the teacher and other school authorities will make it clear to the bullying child and possibly her parents that the behavior is unacceptable. Follow-up with your child to make sure that it does not continue. In addition, work with your child on how to stand up for himself should such an incident happen again. Role-playing self-confident responses, such as ignoring the bully or saying "only people who feel bad about themselves try to hurt other people's feelings," can help a child be prepared the next time.

2. **If your child is in middle school or older, arrange a meeting for your child with the school counselor or other appropriate administrator to discuss the incident(s).** Be present only if your child wants you there. Follow-up with the adult to make sure the meeting occurred. In addition to addressing the bully, hopefully the counselor will help your child develop the skills necessary to confront the bully should it happen again (and you should work with your child on these skills too).

3. **For some preteens or teens it can be difficult to "rat out"' a bully for fear that the bullying will only increase.** If an older child refuses to break the bullying cycle, you may need to watch and wait, as long as your

child is not showing signs of becoming more depressed, demoralized or fearful. However, if it appears that the bullying is getting worse, or your child is really struggling, it may be necessary to intervene no matter how your child feels. A bullied child (even a teen) is an intimidated victim and, therefore, not necessarily the best judge of when to allow a parent to intervene.

4. **If you notice your child becoming less popular due to bullying, or to peers who have withdrawn, it is important to break the cycle and help your child to renew old or establish new friendships.** You may need to be actively involved in arranging activities or play times for your child with other children so that your child doesn't feel isolated and alone.

Negative Force Factor #7:

Pressuring Peers

Sometimes, as a child tries or begins to lose weight, it sets off a strange set of circumstances among his or her friends. Overweight friends can feel jealous that a child is motivated and succeeding. They may try to sabotage the weight loss or even withdraw their friendship in subtle or not so subtle ways because your child's success highlights their own feelings of failure.

Slimmer friends may also feel strangely threatened by a child's new sense of self-confidence or desire to be healthy. In some cases a friendship had been based on the slimmer friend being the more confident or popular one—if this begins to change, the dynamic of the friendship can change too, and your child may find herself the victim of an unexpected jealous backlash.

LAUNCH YOUR ATTACK

1. Explain to your child that although true friendship is based on who you are on the inside and not what you look like on the outside, this is something that children learn as they are growing up and they may not have figured it out just yet.

2. Then point out that perhaps the work to becoming healthier is also making your child more self-confident, have better self-esteem, and feel happier—this could affect friendships positively or negatively.

3. Sometimes, for many different reasons, friendships in childhood go through growing pains and sometimes friendships change altogether. If your child is experiencing this now, you may need to help her negotiate this slightly tough time and choose the friendships that support her healthy lifestyle and changing sense of herself.

4. If necessary, help your child to ask himself the "tough" questions like:

   • Would a real friend treat me like this?

   • Would I treat someone else like this?

   • Why isn't this person happy to see me succeed?

   • What does this tell me about this person?

Negative Force Factor #8:

Style Stressing

Even as young as 7- or 8-year-old children, especially girls, want to fit in with the latest fashions because this is such a big part of fitting in socially. But, when a child is overweight, this can be difficult because so many of the styles are cut for very skinny little bodies. Even boys struggle with this when they're trying to buy a simple pair of jeans. For many over-weight kids, the walk to the fitting room is filled with dread, disguised as an armful of clothing and the walk out is filled with tears and nothing that fits.

Judy (67) tells me about her experience growing up as an overweight child:

> **“**My whole childhood was marked by me being heavy. I could never wear what the other girls wore. My mother bought me ladies clothes and then took up the hems of the pants and the skirts and the sleeves. I always looked terrible. I hated going to school. Sometimes I wished I would just die. If I'd only had fashionable clothes, I think that I would have actually been more motivated to lose weight because I would have felt better about myself from the beginning! Instead, I felt like it was hopeless and that I could never look or feel good, no matter what. It's important for kids to feel good in the clothes they wear, even if they're overweight—feeling good will motivate them to want to take care of their bodies and get healthier and look even better**”**

As Judy explains, in order for children to begin to feel the desire and motivation to lose weight, they must feel good about themselves emotionally. Of course, as they lose weight, they will feel even better about themselves emotionally and physically—the two go hand in hand.

LAUNCH YOUR ATTACK

1. **An important way for a child to feel good is to make sure that they have clothing choices that are fashionable, just as slimmer children do.** This never used to be possible because clothing in larger sizes was never fashionable. But now, thanks to some innovative brands, in a variety of price ranges, launching half sizes and "husky" sizes in many of their styles (even bathing suits), the fashion choices are far greater than they used to be (see Appendix Three for suggestions).

2. **Shop online and let your child try on clothes in the privacy of her own bedroom.** For kids that are stressed by fitting rooms this is an instant anxiety buster. Many stores let you return to the store, even if you purchased online.

3. **Shop with one child at a time, especially if only one is overweight.** Shopping can be especially stressful for an overweight child if a sibling is not having a difficult time finding clothes.

4. **When you take your child shopping, make sure that you focus fully on your child.** Don't allow yourself to become distracted by looking at clothes or other items for yourself or for anyone else.

5. **Accessorize.** Many fashionable accessories for girls and boys (shoes, hats, bandanas, watches, and socks) or other "in" items (pens, chains, earrings, hairclips, etc.) can help a child to feel that he or she fits in. You don't have to go overboard, but perhaps this isn't the time to stand on your principles of "just because everyone else has it, doesn't mean you have to have it!"

❖ ❖ ❖ ❖ ❖

Now that you've conquered the Negative Forces in your child's environment, the next step down the road to your child's good health brings you back into your family to look at habits and patterns that your family might have created. These patterns may have contributed to your child gaining weight to begin with and now they could be getting in the way of your child losing weight. Curious what I'm talking about? Well, turn the page and find out!

Predictable family Patterns

Facing Your Family's Flaws

for many families, struggles with food, weight, and exercise become patterns that seem difficult to change. In fact, sometimes a family pattern may have begun one or more generations before your child was even born. You may not even realize that you are passing down this unhealthy family pattern. If it's all you've known, you may not even know that it's not healthy!

For example, Alexandra, a mom of two, grew up surrounded by a large Italian family in which every meal was an event and every portion was large enough for at least three people. Her grandmother, the matriarch of the family, ruled with an iron spoon, expecting everyone to eat, eat, eat—which they did. As an adult, Alexandra finds herself doing exactly the same thing with her children, Nicole (8) and Mario, Jr. (6). As you might imagine Nicole and Mario have, as a result, both become significantly overweight.

Of course, not all family patterns began in prior generations. Some patterns begin for the first time within your own family. So, in this chapter

I will discuss seven family patterns, giving you exactly the tools you need to recreate healthier patterns for this and future generations.

For each pattern, you will first take a short quiz, to determine whether your family may fit the pattern. Even if you don't fit it exactly, don't skip the section because you will still find thoughts, ideas, and tips that will help you understand your family better.

Pattern #1: Clean Your Plate

Take the Quiz

Answer yes or no to the questions below.

- Do you ask your child frequently if he is hungry?

  YES **NO**

- Is it expected that everyone will have at least "seconds" at every meal, maybe "thirds"?

  YES **NO**

- Do you become upset/hurt/angry/insulted if your child doesn't eat everything on the plate?

  YES **NO**

- Is there always a snack or meal offered in your home long before anyone could ever really, truly be hungry?

  YES **NO**

- Are there always leftovers in the refrigerator because there is always too much food cooked for meals?

  YES **NO**

WHAT YOUR SCORE MEANS

If you answered "yes" to two or more questions there is a very good chance that you are raising your children in a **clean your plate** family—and you may have grown up in one yourself. Even if you answered "yes" to one question you will probably find this section useful.

Aha, Now I Understand

Until Alexandra and her husband Mario came to see me, they didn't realize that the way they were overfeeding their children was actually part of the **clean your plate** pattern, which was contributing to their children becoming and staying overweight.

Sometimes children eats snacks or meals because these are offered, rather than because they are actually hungry. Other times children will eat because they are told to eat by a parent or other adult. Still other times a child will eat because the child knows or senses that an adult will become upset or angry if she doesn't eat. But, when a child eats for any of these reasons, rather than because he is actually *hungry*, the child *stops paying attention to his body's physical need for food and almost always eats much more than he needs to be healthy.* Of course, if a child (or anyone) eats more than his body needs, the result will be an overweight child.

Like Alexandra, many of you reading this book have belonged to the "clean plate club" your whole lives—it might be all you've ever known. You finished your meal because if you didn't it was wrapped in plastic and you were expected to eat it later; or you were told that the starving children in China/India/Africa would be grateful for food as good as this or that your couldn't have dessert if you didn't eat everything on your plate. Or perhaps you were overfed, and you overate because your parents remembered what it was like to be so poor that they knew what it felt like to be truly hungry and they never wanted you to experience that feeling. Cleaning your plate may have become your blueprint for how to feed your children—never say no, always offer more and insist on even more.

You can see that although **clean your plate** is a pattern that derives from love and from not wanting to deprive your child, it doesn't teach a child how to recognize whether he is actually hungry because he is never expected to pay attention to what his body is telling him.

When a child is always offered large helpings of food during and in-between meals, there is very little opportunity for him to think about whether he really wants or needs to eat, or whether he should be having a second helping. In fact, it takes about fifteen minutes for one's brain to register that the stomach has had a satisfying amount of food. If a second helping is already on the plate and being eaten before the fifteen minutes are up, extra calories are being eaten before your child's brain has had a chance to even register the first helping!

Breaking the Pattern

The way to break this pattern is to help your child learn what real hunger feels like and then resist the urge to over-feed your child. You can do so easily by taking the following steps. It may take some practice, but you can do it!

STEP ONE: Jump right to Chapters Six and Seven and start to read the sections about healthy portion sizes for all foods, including the ones you cook and those you eat when you're out.

STEP TWO: Using Chapter Six as your guideline for what portions for foods should be, start serving your child smaller portions for first helpings.

STEP THREE: Don't offer a second helping. This might be tough for you at first, but it'll get easier! If your child asks for seconds, make the second helping half as big as the first helping—except for green salad (with low-fat or no dressing) and veggies (steamed or stir-fried lightly, with a little oil instead of butter or cheesy toppings), these are unlimited.

STEP FOUR: After seconds, tell your child the rule is he must wait fifteen minutes. If he's still hungry he can come back for a piece of fruit. Most kids will have forgotten their "hunger" by then and moved on to something else.

STEP FIVE: Congratulations—you're no longer a clean your plate family!

Pattern #2: Forbidden Foods

Take the Quiz

- Have you forbidden all junk food from your home?

    YES   **NO**

- If there is junk food in your home, do you catch your kids eating it secretly in their rooms, or have you found empty, wrappers hidden around the house?

    YES   **NO**

- Is there mostly "diet," "fat-free," "no-calorie" food in your home?

    YES   **NO**

- Do you sometimes sneak junk food when you think your kids aren't looking?

    YES   **NO**

- Do your kids eat as much junk food as they can at friends' houses, birthday parties or other occasions and then act guiltily when you find out about it?

    YES   **NO**

- Do you have a no junk food rule, but your kids still struggle with their weight?

  YES   **NO**

What Your Score Means

If you answered "yes" to one or more of these questions you may be living in a **forbidden foods** family. Since this type of pattern is the one most likely to be a possible trigger for an eating disorder, it's very important to take a careful look at your family's habits.

Aha, Now I Understand

When Michael, father to Lindsay, Jared, and Jack took this quiz he quickly recognized that he had created a **forbidden foods** home, but he admitted that it had taken him a while to get to that point.

He told me with some embarrassment that when he had divorced two years earlier he had vowed to have a healthier home, and he thought that meant needing to banish all junk food. When his children started bringing secret stashes of candy bars, bags of chips, and gum to their weekends with him, and then hiding the empty wrappers in the closet he became angry with them and with their mother. But taking the quiz and learning about the **forbidden foods** pattern made him realize that rather than being angry with his kids, he needed to find a better approach to helping his children become healthier. Forbidding all junk food wasn't stopping them from eating it, it was just pushing them to do it secretly and that wasn't the kind of relationship he wanted to have with his children.

Try this experiment: Think of your favorite food and then imagine never being able to eat it ever again. What's your first instinct? Of course it's to think about it obsessively and to go and get it right away and eat it! Even as an adult, it's impossible to imagine being told that you can never again eat the foods that you love.

When you raise your child in a **forbidden foods** home, severely limiting the type and the amount of snack or junk foods they are allowed to eat, they crave those foods and very often go to great lengths to get them. In many cases children sneak food that is available when you're not around; binge (overeat) on it when it is available and eat excessive amounts of it when they are at other people's homes. The truth is that many kids gain more weight like this than they would if they had some controlled access to snack foods.

Is this your child? Warning signs that you may have a **forbidden foods** family.

Margaret: I caught Lydia (8) red-handed stuffing her face with birthday cake when she thought no one was looking.

Delores: I found out that Johnny (11) trades his lunch every day for another kid's cookies and chocolate milk!

Tyrone: Shani (10) has been using her lunch money to buy soda and a cookie most days at lunch time—I didn't even know they had a soda machine in school.

Charlene: Every time I send my kids (7 and 10) to sleepovers I tell them not to eat junk food. But one of the moms asked me recently if I knew how much Courtney (7) loves cookies—she ate twelve at one time, watching a movie!

Greg: My wife and I kept a secret tub of ice-cream in the basement freezer that we didn't think the kids knew about until one day I went to get some and it was empty!

In some cases, a child's perception of "forbidden" is different than a parents' idea. Children often feel that a parent is being more restrictive than a parent feels he or she is being and often a negotiation between parent and child becomes important so that the child no longer has the feeling of it being a **forbidden foods** family.

The two biggest concerns that can arise from severely limiting a child's access to the foods they, like all of us, desire are:

1. By not providing them any opportunity to learn how to eat controlled amounts of "junk" food, they will only learn how to eat these foods in sneaky ways, in large amounts, and stuffing their faces, when they get a chance. This will become their blueprint for how to eat junk food. It will be a blueprint they will carry into adulthood.

2. Always feeling the need to sneak the foods they crave and lie to you about it will cause stress, guilt, and shame for your child. This can not only interfere with you and your child developing a close and trusting relationship, it can also become the seeds for your child developing an eating disorder (see Chapter Eight).

Breaking the Pattern

Even though a junk free home is something you've become used to, you can probably see that banishing all junk food from your child's life is actually contributing to your child's struggles with weight by making him crave it, sneak it, and binge on it. So, how do you let a little junk food in without losing total control over your healthy home? Take the following steps and you'll figure it out.

STEP ONE: Although it may be difficult for you initially, the first step to breaking the **forbidden foods** cycle is to bring some snack food or "junk" food into your home. Don't worry, it won't automatically cause your child to gain more weight or make it impossible for him or her to lose weight. Check out Chapter Six for some ideas and consider choices such as baked potato chips, pretzels, granola bars, low-fat cereals, bite size candy bars, unbuttered popcorn, sweetened rice cakes, and small size cookies. Ask your child what snacks he or she really would love to have at home or for school lunches and purchase those.

STEP TWO: Purchase snacks in single serving sizes or immediately repack them into single serving portions (e.g., two cookies, a snack-bag of pretzels), so that your child can immediately begin to see what a serving size looks like and begin practicing the skill of portion controlled eating (lesson #1 in independent healthy eating). **Note that many "single serving" packages of cookies, often purchased in bulk at warehouse supermarkets are really much more than one serving, so read labels carefully.** Chapter Six will teach you about serving sizes and portion control.

STEP THREE. Talk to your child about how many "junk" food snacks he is allowed each day—one is usually enough. For an older child (about ten years old or above, you might consider two if it becomes a battle of wills). Allow your child to decide if he would like the snack(s) for school lunch or at home after school or after dinner. Giving your child this choice is lesson #2 in independent healthy eating.

STEP FOUR: When your child goes to someone else's home, or to a party, discuss realistic eating goals but don't forbid junk food eating. Remember, this is a process for you and for your child. Your goal is to reduce and eventually eliminate the secrets, the guilt, and also the overeating and binge eating. If this doesn't seem to be happening, read Chapter Eight carefully.

Pattern #3: Snacking Is Sweeter

Take the Quiz

- Are your kitchen cabinets filled with a large variety of every kind of snack food?

    YES   **NO**

- Are meals generally a second thought in your family, because no one is really hungry since they've been snacking throughout the day?

    YES   **NO**

- Is the refrigerator mostly empty because preparing meals and cooking don't happen very often in your home?

    YES   **NO**

- Is it easy for your kids to grab a soda, glass of juice or other sugar-sweetened drink whenever they want one?

    YES   **NO**

- Do you, or your child's other primary caretaker (babysitter, grandparent), rarely say "no" to snacking, no matter what time of day it is?

    YES   **NO**

WHAT YOUR SCORE MEANS

If you responded "yes" to one or more questions, you're probably living in a **snacking is sweeter** family. Since snacking is one of the main reasons that kids become overweight, it's time to understand what this means for your children!

Aha, Now I Understand

Nancy and Rick both work full-time—Nancy is an accountant and Rick owns a small construction company. They log many work hours a week and have a full-time babysitter, Konnie, taking care of their kids, Daniella (6) and Charlotte (3). They feel fortunate because Konnie adores the girls. However, she will not refuse them ANYTHING, including whatever they want to eat and Daniella and Charlotte are both now officially overweight according to their doctor.

In the evenings and on weekends, Nancy and Rick also find it difficult to say "no" to the girls because they don't want to ruin their precious time together with temper tantrums and meltdowns. But both parents know the doctor is right—something must change—their daughters' physical and emotional health are at terrible risk!

In some families snacking on high-calorie, high-fat, sugary foods, candy, treats, crackers, cereals, cookies, puddings, cupcakes, and drinks is a common occurrence and can happen for many reasons. Do any of these sound familiar to you?

Esther: My kids nag and nag and never stop. I can't stand it so I just give in—it's easier than the nagging.

Courtney: My husband and I disagree about the snacking. He thinks they should be able to have whatever they want because they're just kids. I think they should have one or two snacks a day. But I don't want to fight with him, so I let them eat what they want or they go running to daddy.

Steven: I'm a stay at home dad and I always feel like I'm being judged by the moms if my kids cry, so I probably give in a little too often to keep them smiling.

Lashaunda: I'm divorced and their dad gives them whatever they want. I don't want to be the bad guy all the time, so I let them have the junk food they ask for.

Harriet: After working a full week, I want to enjoy my children. They're so happy when I let them have the snacks they want—what's the big deal? I'll deal with their weight when they're older.

Felipe: Admittedly, we all like to snack, not just the kids. It would be impossible to take the junk food out of the house because the adults eat it all day long too.

Louise: I couldn't live without junk food all day long—it's how I bribe my kids to do what I want them to do!

As you can see you're not alone when it comes to being a **snacking is sweeter** family. But when children eat too many snacks throughout the day, they are not hungry for healthy meals and they also consume *far too many calories and easily become overweight.*

In addition, as with **clean your plate**, if a child is always snacking, he or she won't learn to pay attention to hunger cues or recognize the feeling of being satisfied. *Too much snacking is one of the top reasons children gain weight and don't lose it.*

Breaking the Pattern

As you can probably tell from the above parents' stories, there's a lot more to **snacking is sweeter** than just letting your children eat too many snacks. There are several reasons that parents allow their children to snack too much. These are listed on the left side of the table below. Which one (or more) fits your family?

On the right side of the table is the way to begin addressing each reason. Identifying and addressing each of these is **STEP ONE** in breaking the **snacking is sweeter** pattern. Steps two through five are below.

Your Family's Reason	The Change You Should Make
I'm not strong enough to say "NO" when my child asks, demands, then tantrums for a snack. I give in because I can't stand the whining or screaming or because she's embarrassing me in public.	Begin to say "NO" when it's not snack time. Don't be afraid of a tantrum–no child was ever hurt by one! It will only take a few times of saying "NO" and sticking to it, for your child to get the message. Your child's health is worth it.
I have a child-care provider that does things the way she wants to–and I can't seem to change it. I've asked, but I'm either ignored or she changes her ways only for a day or two.	It's time to be the boss and the parent. Even a wonderful babysitter (or grandparent) needs to be taught the new snacking rules. If necessary write them down. If you must, keep all snacks, except those for the day locked up so the babysitter isn't tempted to give in to your child.
I don't know which snacks are healthy and which aren't; I don't know how many snacks a day is healthy for my child to be eating.	Read Chapter Six carefully. You will learn everything you need to know about healthy snacking.
I disagree with my child's other parent (married or divorced) about healthy snacking. One of us thinks that it's okay for a child to have as many snacks during the day as they want and the other one thinks there should be restrictions.	If you are married, you and your partner should discuss your child's health together–reading this book as a team will help. If you are divorced, you only have control over your home. Do your best to teach your child about healthy snacking. Perhaps a trip to the doctor with your child would convince his other parent that healthier eating is in order.

Your Family's Reason	The Change You Should Make
The whole family eats too much junk food so it would be hard to get rid of it in our home.	Read Chapter Six—there's no need to eliminate junk food from your family's life all together. Rather, it's time to reduce the amount of snack food you have at home and substitute it for healthier snack foods. I'm confident you'll find that your child's physical and emotional health is worth the changes you'll need to make!
I use junk food to get my kids to behave compliantly (e.g., if you clean up your toys/do your homework/stop fighting/ put away your laundry/then you can have a lollipop/cookie/ice cream/soda.	Immediately replace food snacks with another form of incentive. If you have a difficult time motivating your child to behave well, take a good parent- ing class at your child's school or lo- cal library. You're sure to learn some great skills!

STEP TWO: Read Chapter Six to learn about the healthiest snacks to have in your home. Some ideas to consid- er are baked potato chips, yogurt, fruit, pretzels, unbuttered popcorn, dried fruit, granola bars, low-fat cereals, bite size candy bars, sweetened rice cakes, and small size cookies.

STEP THREE: This step and the next one are exactly the same as two of the steps in the **Forbidden Foods** pattern. This is because there are similarities be- tween patterns and many families struggle with more than one pattern.

Purchase snacks in single serving sizes or immediately repack them into single serving portions (e.g., two cookies, a snack bag of pretzels), so that your child can immediately begin to see what a serving size looks like and begin practicing the skill of portion-controlled eating (lesson #1 in independent healthy eating). **Note that many "single serving" packages of cookies, often purchased in bulk at warehouse supermarkets, are really much more than one serving, so read labels carefully.** Chapter Six will teach you about serving sizes and portion control.

STEP FOUR: Talk to your child about how many "junk" food snacks he is allowed each day—one is usually enough. For an older child (about ten years old or above, you might consider two if it becomes a battle of wills). Allow your child to decide if he would like the snack(s) for school lunch or at home after school or after dinner. Giving your child this choice is lesson #2 in independent healthy eating.

STEP FIVE: Be prepared to have healthy meals prepared for your child. Once you've reduced the high calorie, between meal snacking, your child will begin to learn what it feels like to be hungry and you need to be ready with the right food.

Pattern #4: Fast Living, Fast Food

Take the Quiz

- Do your children eat almost all meals on the run?

  YES   **NO**

- Are your children's meals usually from a drive-thru?

  YES   **NO**

73

- Do you usually feed your children whatever is fastest and most convenient, rather than focusing on what is healthiest?

    YES   **NO**

- Is your refrigerator mostly empty because no one really cooks in your home?

    YES   **NO**

What Your Score Means

If you answered "yes" to two or more questions, it's likely that you are in a **fast living, fast food** family, but even one "yes" probably means you should be making some changes, so read on!

Aha, Now I Understand

Cindy is a single mom juggling Kylie (10), two jobs, a house, a dog, and two hamsters. "Sometimes, it's all I can do to drag myself out of bed in the morning and get Kylie up for school," admitted Cindy. "I know that feeding Kylie fast food all the time isn't good for her. I can see that she's gained a lot of weight and that she's not happy about it, but I just don't have a single minute left in the day to cook!"

Cindy is not alone living in her intensely-paced world, which leaves little time to breathe, let alone cook. To make it worse, fast-food companies inundate our children and us with enticing advertising and "great deals," to purchase their high-calorie, high fat, not very nutritious products. No wonder **fast living, fast food** is making our kids gain weight (and sometimes us too!).

Breaking the Pattern

Believe it or not, I'm **not** going to tell you that you have to stop eating fast food! The truth is that just about every fast food restaurant now has healthier choices on the menu. Your job will be getting your child to eat them—*that* might be a bit tricky.

STEP ONE: Begin by downsizing. The extra-large, double, supersized whatever your child normally orders, is TOO BIG! So wherever you go, explain to your child that from now on you'll be ordering either kid-size or regular sized burgers, fries or nuggets. Since your child may be used to eating more food, you can supplement with fresh fruit (some fast-food places sell fruit, otherwise bring it with you). Also, always order water or seltzer—not soda!

Next, many fast-food restaurants have healthier choices on the menu, so if your child will try these, they're always a better option. In order to make sure that you're making all the best fast-food choices for your child, take a look at the complete list of suggestions in Chapter Seven. Read all the categories that apply to the types of fast food restaurants that your family is likely to frequent for breakfast, lunch, and dinner.

STEP TWO: Put your fridge to good use and start stocking healthy "fast food" at home. Talk to your kids about what foods they like and look for the healthy versions of these. See Chapters Six and Seven for lots of ideas. An added bonus is that it will cost you a lot less to eat out less often. For example, yogurt, string cheese, fruit, low-fat deli meats and low-fat hot dogs are all super-quick to make and much healthier than eating at fast-food restaurants.

Breakfast is an especially good time to focus on healthier fast food because you're probably at home already. Here are a couple of easy ideas:

- A bowl of high fiber cereal with low-fat or fat-free milk is quick and healthy

- A slice of whole wheat or multigrain bread with peanut-butter

- A string cheese and an apple

- A low-fat yogurt and a cut-up orange

- A low-fat granola bar and a glass of fat-free milk

I'd love to hear the super-quick, healthy breakfasts that your kids love. I'll share them with other readers. Email them to me at quickandhealthy@ kidsonlyweightloss.com.

Pattern #5: Sibling Stress

Take the Quiz

- Do you have one child that is overweight and another that is average or even underweight?

    YES   **NO**

- Does your overweight child become easily angry with, mean to, or jealous of your slimmer child?

    YES   **NO**

- Do you sometimes become frustrated with your over-weight child or think that, compared to your slimmer child, she isn't trying hard enough to take the necessary steps to lose weight?

    YES   **NO**

- Does your overweight child compare himself negatively to your slimmer child?

  YES   **NO**

- Does your overweight child believe that you favor your slimmer child when it comes to food?

  YES   **NO**

WHAT YOUR SCORE MEANS

If you responded "yes" to two or more questions, your children might be experiencing the pattern of **sibling stress**. Since enjoying a positive sibling relationship is critical for all children, taking the time to understand and break this pattern will be important for them.

Aha, Now I Understand

When it comes to food, Danny (12) always feels that his younger brother Noah (10) gets the better deal. "And maybe he's right," acknowledges, the boys' father, George. The doctor has told us that Danny needs to lose weight. So when we go for pizza, Danny gets one slice and a salad. But Noah is skinny, why shouldn't he have a second slice? Danny gets crazy, though— but doesn't he want to be thinner, like Noah?"

A small amount of rivalry is a natural part of all sibling relationships, but when it takes over, causing jealousy, anger, and constant fighting it isn't healthy for either child. In some cases, as with George, parents fuel the **sibling stress** without even realizing that they are doing so.

Breaking the Pattern

In order to break the **sibling stress** pattern, follow the Seven Sibling Stress Relievers tips on the list below.

- At home or in a restaurant, all siblings should be offered the same choices—a slimmer child doesn't need *more* of unhealthy food any more than an overweight child needs it.

- Refrain from comparing children—there is **never** a time when this is useful, motivating or has a positive outcome, no matter what your reason for doing it.

- Go clothing shopping separately with siblings (boys and girls)—trying on clothes is stressful for overweight kids. It's much worse when a slim sibling looks great in everything. Even better, shop online, one child at a time. Several companies now make clothing lines for overweight kids. See Appendix Three for some suggestions.

- Become aware of feelings you may have about blaming your overweight child for not eating healthily or exercising compared to your slimmer child. It is important not to verbalize these feelings to any of your children. It is also critical to recognize that *your child needs your help* to become healthier—no child can do it alone!

- Jealousy is not an excuse to treat a sibling badly. If your overweight child is mean to a sibling, speak to her privately. Your child may not even realize that her jealousy is driving the poor behavior. You can gently make the connection and then explain that the behavior is not acceptable. Yelling or punishing will not help in this case and may only worsen the jealousy or anger.

- A slimmer sibling must be made clearly aware that teasing, taunting, and name-calling about weight are unacceptable. Such comments, even in jest can have long-term damaging effects on an overweight child's self-esteem and body-image, especially when made by a close family member.

- Talk to your overweight child about his feelings. Acknowledge that it is hard to have a slimmer sibling. Then, with your child, make a list of all his wonderful traits that have nothing to do with weight.

Pattern #6: Electronics versus Exercise

Take the Quiz

- Do your children spend much of their free time watching TV and playing on the computer and video games?

    YES   **NO**

- Are the bikes, jump ropes, hula hoops, skateboards, roller skates, ice-skates gathering dust in the garage most of the year?

    YES   **NO**

- Are most of your child's extra-curricular activities sedentary (e.g., music lessons, art) rather than active (sports, dance)?

    YES   **NO**

WHAT YOUR SCORE MEANS

If you answered "yes" to any of the above questions, you and your children are probably members of an **electronics versus exercise** family. Since we live in a world so dominated by TV and electronics, it's easy for children to become couch potatoes (and us too!). But, it's not good for their physical or psychological health. Read on to find out how to get your child moving without kicking and screaming!

Aha, Now I Understand

Lydia acknowledges her plight: "We have four kids ranging in age from three to fourteen. Although I know I should be getting them out more, playing ball and riding bikes, it's just so much easier to let the TV and computer occupy them while I make dinner, or my husband is paying bills or doing homework with one child."

It is tempting to allow the electronics in our homes to baby-sit our kids—it's so peaceful! And to tell you the truth, I see nothing wrong with a little peace and quiet that a good TV show can bring to a chaotic home at the end of the day.

But research shows us that one of the clear reasons for children's weight gain throughout the western world is that children are becoming more and more sedentary with each generation. It's not hard to see that along with motorized transportation, TV and all other electronics are the reason for this. The less a child moves, the fewer calories from food are expended for energy. Instead, that food is simply converted into fat.

Breaking the Pattern

I would never suggest that you take away the TV or the electronics—you might come after me and throw this book at me! But, there are some things you absolutely can and should do that will break the **electronics versus exercise** pattern and jumpstart your child.

STEP ONE: Limit the TV and electronics. There's no need to tell your child that this is for health reasons (they'll throw the book at you). Rather, *all* families should have a weeknight rule that says "NO TV or electronics until all homework, dinner, chores, and showers are finished." You simply need to add "30 minutes of play time." to the list. If you don't already have this rule, *it's time that you made it!!* If it's a nice day you can insist that they play outside. This will automatically make the play more active. But even inside play—even a board game—is more kinetic than the TV! For many children, the thirty minutes will be so much fun that they will naturally extend it.

STEP TWO: Make another rule that says "No food while watching TV (even during meals), or playing with electronics." If it's easier for you, make a "No eating in the den/living room/at the desk/computer table/on the couch" rule too. Eating while being sedentary is another of the reasons that sedentary kids gain weight. It's worth re-reading Chapter Three to remind you about the way the media impacts weight gain in children.

STEP THREE: When you're ready to really get your child moving, head over to Chapter Nine to learn some more tips and tricks for sneaking exercise into your child's daily life. You'll even learn how to use TV time to become exercise time. If you're really curious, take a look right now, but don't forget to come back here.

Pattern #7: Food Equals Love

Take the Quiz

- Did you grow up in a family in which food was the focus of all events whether celebratory or sad?

  YES   NO

- Is food at the heart of most or all of your family's events, parties, celebrations, and get-togethers?

  YES   **NO**

- Is food used in your family to express positive feelings (for example, grandparents who cook extra-large meals; parents who express love by giving a food "treat" or who return from work or vacation with candy)?

  YES   **NO**

- Do you find it easy to use food as means of comfort or to relieve your child's emotional pain—either deliberately or without realizing it at the time?

  YES   **NO**

WHAT YOUR SCORE MEANS

If you answered "yes" to one or more of the above questions, then it is likely that you live in a **food equals love** family. In many cases, this was the type of family in which you grew up—in fact, to reject food may have meant you were rejecting your parent's love. But it is time to break this cycle and create a new one in which love does not rely on food for its expression.

Aha, Now I Understand

Peter, one of the parents in my Parent Advisory Group, shared the poignant and powerful expression of his **food equals love** life experience.

"For all the reasons you can possibly imagine, I have offered food as comfort, as solace, as tribute, as love. It was the heart of all our celebrations and the center of our time together as family. Extra sweet, extra rich, extra generous . . . food was what I offered to show my family I cared for them. I have changed in the past year and hope to show my family my love in healthier ways."

I am grateful to Peter for allowing me to share his honest, and I imagine sometimes soul-searching journey, toward his family's health. Like Peter, many parents use food to express love and unwittingly undermine their children's good health by doing this. So, as you can see you are not alone and you too can find healthier ways to show love for *your* family.

Breaking the Pattern

Your goal is to learn how to express love toward your child without relying on food to do so. However, if your family's **food equals love** pattern extends to more than just your immediate family, it may be frustrating because you feel that you are being thwarted at every turn by grandparents, aunts, uncles, and cousins. And admittedly it is difficult, and often impossible to change everyone in your extended family. But don't be disconcerted. It is most important to make changes in your immediate family's eating patterns—within your household. This is where your child spends most of the time.

Of course, if your child spends a significant amount of time with other relatives, you will have to talk to them too—even offer this book to them. If they are not receptive to making healthy changes to help your child, you may have to consider how much time your child spends with this family member. Of course, this is not always simple, especially if you rely on a grandparent or other relative for child care. But first, begin at home because you can't expect other people to make changes for your child if you haven't done so first. So, follow the two steps below to break the **food equals love** pattern.

STEP ONE: In order to help you begin thinking about your feelings of love for your child instead of simply reacting to them by offering food, I will ask you to write about two different topics.

The first is a description of your love for your child and what these feelings are like for you. Use as many descriptive words as you can and really try and get in touch with your own feelings about your child. Try and write as much as you can, and don't worry about how well it is written, whether or not it is grammatically correct or if there are misspelled words. You don't need to show anyone what you have written (but you can if you want to).

Second, write a story about how you use food to express love to your child. If you grew up in a family that used food to express love, include this in your story. Describe the circumstances in which you might find yourself offering food to show your love, list the foods that you usually offer, and describe the way it makes you feel to see your child eat the food that you have provided out of love.

STEP TWO: Reread your stories a few times over several days and then ask yourself this important question: What are nonfood ways that you can employ that will give you the same feelings you wrote about in Step one?

Below are some examples that have worked for many families. I'd love to share your ideas with other parents. You can email them to me at DrSusan@kidsonlyweightloss.com.

- Writing in journal together

- Scrapbooking together

- Playing a board game as a family

- Creating a family quilt

- Beginning a nonfood family tradition, such as a scavenger hunt or soccer game

- Offering nonfood gifts for your child

❧ ❧ ❧ ❧ ❧

You've covered a lot of ground now, learning the seven family patterns and you're well on your way to really helping your child become healthier. The next big step is to understand how your child's—and even your own—feelings cause your child to gain or not lose weight. Take a look at Chapter Five and let's keep going!

Feelings can Make a child fat

The Food-Mood Connection

Many (maybe even most) people—adults and children alike—eat not just to satisfy a biological need. Rather they eat to gratify or assuage one or more of the feelings that they experience each day. People eat when they are happy, sad, angry, disappointed, nervous, excited, moody, tired, relieved, worried, anxious, bored, joyful, depressed, lazy, melancholy, tense, and every feeling in between.

Children that are overweight often do this more and perhaps as more of a crutch, than those that are not overweight. It is important to understand how a child develops this crutch and what you, as a parent can do to reduce or eliminate the need for it.

Think about which feelings trigger you to eat. Parents are role models for their children in many ways, including in establishing eating habits. So, if *you* eat to express or manage your feelings, there's a good chance your children do too. Think about the following questions and answer them honestly.

- If you come home from work stressed and in a bad mood do you grab a bag of chips (or other snack)?

  YES   **NO**

- When you're feeling sad or down, do you turn to cookies, ice-cream or other comfort food cheer you up?

  YES   **NO**

- When you have a personal or professional success do you almost always celebrate with food?

  YES   **NO**

- When you have nothing else to do, do you turn to food to occupy you?

  YES   **NO**

- Do you eat when you're worried, anxious or nervous?

  YES   **NO**

- Is eating something you do to boost your energy when you're tired or lethargic?

  YES   **NO**

The Kid Connection

If you answered "Yes" to any of these questions, it means that you may use food as a way to express or manage your feelings and it's very likely that you're communicating this message to your child. Even without even realizing it, you're probably encouraging your child to use food to express or manage his or her feelings. So, now, answer the following questions to help you figure it out.

- If your child comes home from school upset, do you offer a cookie or other snack to cheer him up?

    YES   **NO**

- When your child has an accomplishment do you go out for pizza or another type of celebratory meal?

    YES   **NO**

- If your child is feeling down because she had a fight with her best friend do you suggest an ice-cream cone to cheer her up?

    YES   **NO**

- Is food the main focus of every birthday party?

    YES   **NO**

- Does your child turn to food when he is bored?

    YES   **NO**

- Do you sometimes bribe your child to behave better, calm down, relax, be less angry, stop yelling or be polite, by offering a (junk) food reward?

    YES   **NO**

If you answered "Yes" to any of the above questions it may mean that you are teaching your child to use food as strategy for coping with, or expressing, feelings. The more times you answered "Yes" the more likely it is that you are doing so. By encouraging your child to use food to manage feelings, even by teaching this, you are thwarting opportunities for your child to really confront and work through a wide range of both positive and negative feelings in many different circumstances. Instead, your child will begin to use food as a crutch when she is feeling sad, angry or anxious. Food will become the focus of every celebration. Food will also be the way your child soothes herself during times of stress. When food becomes the manner in which your child manages many important emotions and emotionally charged life situations, it is easy to see how overeating and weight gain can become a significant issue for a child.

Break the Cycle

In order to help your child learn how to stop using food to manage feelings, you're going to need to make some changes yourself! These won't be difficult, but they will take some getting used to. Take the following steps and before long you'll notice a huge difference in your family.

STEP ONE: Write a list of all the times that food is an *unnecessary* factor in your child's life. Look to the quiz above for ideas as to when this may be. In addition, think carefully of other times it may be happening. Food may be playing a much more complex role in your child's emotional life than you realize. Some other examples when you may be allowing food to satisfy an emotional need for your child include:

- Distracting an anxious or angry child with a food treat.

- Offering a sugary snack to a tired child in need of an energy boost.

- A random "family tradition" that's not attached to any real tradition just because it makes everyone happy (e.g., every Sunday night we go out for pizza; the first Thursday of the month is the "All you can eat Chinese buffet").

- Making food and eating the center of play time with a friend because it's easier to see kids smiling than to see them bored or frustrated.

- Having too much food at a party (everyone should have enough party food, excessive party food sends the wrong message–especially if you keep the leftovers).

STEP TWO: Think of and write down appropriate nonfood substitutes for each example on your list. This step may take more than a couple of minutes. In fact, if you've been relying on food to manage many feelings for much of your, as well as your child's life, it may even take you a few days or weeks, to really come up with great substitutions, but it'll be worth it! Your child, with your help, needs to learn that food cannot hold such a powerful role in his life. Feelings need to be experienced and to be managed healthily–not to be stuffed down or washed away with food. Some examples include:

- Playing a game of cards as a distraction when your child is angry or anxious instead of using food.

- Suggesting a bike ride for an energy boost, instead of a sugary snack.

- Creating a new family tradition (for example, a football game or a garage sale).

STEP THREE: Work toward using all the nonfood substitutions that you've come up with. Keep your list handy all the time and review it daily so you get used to your new nonfood way of thinking. I bet you'll find that it helps not only your child's eating, but your own as well!

The Feelings Factor

Now that you understand how you and your child's feelings can make your child eat more and possibly become overweight, it is also valuable look at how your feelings *about* your child's weight could be contributing to your child being overweight.

There are five feelings that you could be experiencing that, each in its own way, may impact your child and might even be contributing to her weight and body image struggles. These feelings are **Fear, Shame, Anger, Guilt,** and **Frustration**.

Fear and a Quick Fix

For many parents, **Fear** plays a significant role in how they choose to manage an overweight child. You may be fearful that your child is being teased; you could be afraid that he is destined for a life of heartbreak; your fear could be about your child's physical health; or perhaps you are fearful that your child will suffer the same struggles that you experienced as a child or adult.

Your fear could come from any number of places, but many parents try to alleviate their fear by trying to quickly "fix" their child's problem by controlling every aspect of their child's eating life in the hope that their child will quickly lose weight and no longer have the weight problem that is causing both child and parent so much anxiety.

Many teens I speak with describe their "fixing" parents as "control freaks who don't ever trust me to even try to make the right eating decision!"

Jordana (14) described her mother as follows: "She sits in the living room and listens to every sound I make in the kitchen. When she hears the door to the snack cupboard opening, she walks into the kitchen pretending she's come in for something else. Really she wants to make sure I'm not going to eat something that she thinks is bad for me! But I've figured it out—I hide it under my sweatshirt, sneak it up to my room and eat there."

As with Jordana, your fear and subsequent attempt to quickly fix your child's eating habits will backfire and cause your child to eat secretly when you're not around (if you're not sure about this, read Chapter Four, Pattern #2: Forbidden Foods).

The Fear of Fat

For many parents—more often mothers—their own fear of becoming overweight, and constantly worrying that they are fat, is communicated to a child or teen without the parent even realizing it. This message can result in that youngster worrying excessively about her own weight or body image. It can also lead to secret or closet eating, which can result in a child becoming overweight or developing an eating disorder (or both).

Take the following quiz to see whether you may be communicating too many weight fears to your daughter or son.

1. Do you weigh yourself more than once a month in front of your child?

2. When the family eats meals together, do you tend to pick at your food, rather than enjoying the meal with everyone else?

3. Does exercise take precedence over almost every other activity in your life?

4. Do you talk in front of your child about dieting, watching your weight, losing weight or how fat you think you are (you may need to ask someone else to give you an objective answer to this question)?

5. Are you almost always dissatisfied with the way you look in clothes and do you express this openly?

6. Do you put your body down in front of your child?

If you answered "yes" to any one, and certainly to more, of the above questions, you could be giving your child the message that you are not satisfied with your body and that it is unlikely that, no matter how much you try, you ever will be.

In addition, you are also letting your child know that you are so fearful of being overweight that you will go to extremes such as overexercising, overweighing, undereating, and/or over-obsessing, in order to keep your weight and that fear in check.

I'm sure that now I've explained the strong connection between fear and your child's weight, you want to begin to make changes in the behavior that you are role modeling for your child, so that you can give your child every chance possible to not only become healthier, but also to reduce any possibility that she will develop an eating disorder. But, if you have any concern that your child is exhibiting signs of an eating disorder, take a look at Chapter Eight.

Fixing Your Fear

Instead of letting your fear tempt you to try a quick fix, take a deep breath and start to realize that helping your child learn a lifetime of healthy habits and skills is going to be a long-term project. By following the steps in this chapter, you'll find that your fear will naturally diminish because you are doing something productive and practical to help your child. Quick fixes and panic don't work Rather, take slow and steady steps. In addition, explain to your child that becoming healthy is a long-term process. You'll do great!

In addition, the following three simple steps will get you on your way.

STEP ONE: Refrain from weighing yourself in front of your child. Keep the scale hidden so your child can't weigh himself either.

STEP TWO: Don't speak negatively about your own body, the way you look in clothes or any other aspect of yourself in front of your child.

STEP THREE: Try to eat and exercise in moderation. If this is a great struggle for you—hide the struggle from your child. Your child needs to see you eating healthy meals—rather than overeating or skipping meals; exercising regularly—not over or under exercising.

The Secret of Shame

It can be hard to admit, but some parents secretly feel **Shame** that their child is overweight. This can be especially true if you have never struggled with being overweight yourself or if you happen to live in a community where most people are fit or a within a family where being slim is very highly valued. In any one of these situations, it can secretly feel like a burden or embarrassment to have an overweight child. If you have these feelings of shame or embarrassment, you probably don't want to admit them to anyone because parents aren't supposed to be ashamed of their children—right?!

But even if you don't admit it out loud, it is likely that these feelings are bound to affect the way you interact with your child, so it is valuable to address them. The most common reaction that shame elicits from a parent is to try and "hide" their child's body with clothing.

Leslie, mother to Roy (10) and Janna (10), both who are overweight, admitted to feeling ashamed of her children's weight. "I've always been thin," she told me "so how did I let them get so out of control? I try to disguise their bodies with loose fitting clothing and they just get so angry, especially Janna—she says that I'm ashamed of her. I guess she's not wrong. I wish I could feel differently."

When a child (especially a preteen or teen) feels that a parent is overly focused on "flattering clothing" it makes the child angry, uncomfortable, and rejected. This could trigger a child to feel even less motivated to try and lose weight. Tweens and teens in particular, quickly hone in on a parent's shame and embarrassment and become deeply hurt—even scarred into adulthood—by it. In addition, the child may also feel that the parent is focusing on the way she looks on the outside, rather than on the inside. Over time the child or teen may also come to focus primarily on superficial aspects of him or herself, thereby devaluing, and even feeling ashamed of, the far more important core sense of self.

The Shift from Shame

It is critical to be sensitive to your child's struggles not only with weight, but with clothing too. Here are six steps to help you manage your feelings about your child's clothing choices, which will begin to alleviate stress for your child as you work through your feelings of shame.

1. Ask your child how he would like to dress. Do not insist on baggy clothes, simply to satisfy your feeling of shame or embarrassment.

2. Seek compromise with your child to find clothing that fits well (not too tight/not too loose) and that is as fashionable as your child desires and can find at her weight. In addition, compliment her generously when she clearly feels good in an outfit. See Appendix Three for some sources.

3. If clothing shopping is too stressful for you and your child, send your child with his other parent or another adult (grandparent, aunt, friend, etc.). [Note: This may be especially necessary if you are a naturally thin parent shopping with an overweight child of the same gender (especially mothers and daughters).]

4. Refrain from making negative comments about your child's physical appearance in clothing except under extreme circumstances—and even then be very careful about how you communicate. Be as gentle as possible and explain specifically why you're making the comment. Then thank your child for compromising. For example, "That outfit will work fine for school, but it really isn't great to go to a wedding. Do you think you could wear something a bit dressier/ with fewer holes in it/that's not tie-dyed? Thanks, I really appreciate you making the change."

5. Talk to your child about working together as a family to make changes toward a healthier lifestyle. As you read through the book you will find many ways to accomplish this goal.

6. If you struggle considerably with feelings of shame, consider seeking professional, psychological help. Speaking with someone about your feelings may help you identify when your child's behavior "pushes your buttons," as one of the members of my Parents Advisory Group described it, and most importantly, maintain a good relationship with your child.

The Rules for Shopping with an Overweight Child

1. Never tell a child he looks fat in something.

2. Shop with one child in the family at a time—even if both are overweight.

3. Resist the urge to go shopping with your child's friend and her mom—it may sound like fun in theory, but the reality may be upsetting for your child.

4. If you're shopping with a child, preteen, or teen of the same gender as you, *don't* try on clothes together, especially if you're a smaller size—no matter how tempted you may be. Come back another day to shop for yourself.

5. Don't take your child to a clothing store unless you're sure there will be at least a few items that should fit—check the store out first.

6. Shop online—for many children it's much less stressful. Many parents find it much more relaxing as well, and the possibility of needing to manage returns is well worth it if your child's experience is happier. Prepare your child for the possibility that clothing will need to be returned if it doesn't fit or if you

or your child don't like it when you see it "live." Assure your child that returns are no big deal! In addition, many stores have a greater online than in-store selection of plus size clothing (see Appendix Three for sources).

In some cases overweight kids and teens choose to dress and express themselves in wildly unusual ways in order to hide or distract from their overweight bodies. Older teens may color their hair, paint their fingernails crazy colors, and wear unusual hats, scarves, shoes, and other accessories (boys and girls). This can also trigger embarrassment and shame in parents who may not understand the reason for a child's choice of clothing.

Rather than becoming angry with a child for dressing and expressing in an avant garde manner, or even simply in a style that you do not like (as long as it is not sexualized or otherwise inappropriate), it is very important to support your child through this difficult time of life. Look at your child's way of dressing as unique, creative, and artistic. Find ways to help your child feel good about this form of self-expression, because the positive self-esteem you give your child—rather than criticism—may be just what he needs in order to develop the inner strength to work on losing weight.

If you happen to be a more conservative person and find this form of self-expression particularly difficult, keep reminding yourself that in all likelihood it is temporary. It is a time for your child to cope with a current, painful struggle with weight and body image. Children go through many phases during their development. Right now this may seem larger than life to you because it is touching on an area that is eliciting your own feelings of shame. But it is important for you to separate out your feelings from your child's struggle and support your child through this time.

Once your child has other coping strategies, the need to using clothing to express or hide feelings will probably be over. The harder you work to help your child manage feelings more effectively, the less she will need to rely on clothing for that reason. Of course, if your child is naturally artistic, seeing the world through eyes slightly different than the rest of us, and dresses this way for other reasons . . . well then you're on your own. Personally, I admire those kids and adults who can pull it off effectively!

Overwhelming Anger

Anger is another response that parents sometimes feel when they are confronted with an overweight child. You may experience anger because the doctor, spouse or grandparent blames you for the child's weight problem. You may be angry because your child isn't cooperative about eating or exercising the way he should be or simply because you're frustrated about the situation.

Anger about having an overweight child is understandable and can have its root in many places in addition to the ones just mentioned. The problem is that often parents express this anger directly at their overweight child. Arguments ensue about food, exercise or clothing. You may find yourself short-tempered with your child, frustrated, and even inadvertently blaming your child for being overweight.

A recent Stanford Medical Center study, reported in the journal *Pediatrics,* found that many college girls who, as children, had heard negative comments from family members about their weight or shape grew up to have a negative body images and poor self-esteem.

Most remarkable about these results is that the study found even occasional remarks could have a lasting negative effect. In fact, within an otherwise warm, loving family, these type of remarks would stand out as even more hurtful and long-lasting.

Sometimes parents express anger in a slightly veiled way, through sarcasm—which is anger and humor combined. Sarcasm is just as hurtful—sometimes even more so—and just as angry as yelling or insults. Most children and many teens can't respond effectively to sarcasm because they have not yet developed language that is sophisticated enough to do so. They are therefore at a disadvantage when a parent lashes out with a sarcastic, insulting, and always hurtful comment. Sarcastic comments about weight or body shape will hurt just as much as direct anger.

The Paradoxical Effect of Anger

Aside from harming a child's self-esteem, it is very important to realize that yelling, reprimanding, sarcasm, and anger *don't work* to help a child eat more healthily or exercise more frequently. In fact, these responses may even have the opposite effect on your child's behavior. Some members of my Parents Advisory Group shared that when they have become frustrated or angry with their children or made negative comments to them, it has resulted in their kids overeating or refusing to exercise simply to spite their parents. In fact, this is not unusual. Children often respond to anger defensively—as do we all! Defensive feelings frequently result in a child trying to regain control or expressing frustration by refusing to do what he knows you want done.

It is clear to see that by yelling, criticizing or reprimanding your child you could be painting her into a corner, the only way out of which is to blatantly defy you. In many cases, this results in a vicious cycle, infuriating you more, causing more yelling. It's time to end the anger.

Abolish Anger

As you can see, your anger has the potential to result in you saying things you may regret, and that could affect your child far into the future. In addition, anger can actually have the opposite effect than the one you're trying to achieve. It is therefore critical for you to understand and gain control over this complex feeling.

In order to do this you need to separate the love you have for your child from the frustration and anger you have about his weight. This is not always easy to do, but it is so important and can be done by taking the following four steps.

> **STEP ONE:** Make a list of all your child's positive traits, strengths, and qualities. Take your time, make the list as long, detailed, and comprehensive as possible and *write this list down.* Include both big and small things. Making this list will help you see that your child is so much more wonderful and special than just his weight. Keep the list with you and refer to it whenever you start to feel angry.

> **STEP TWO:** When you're feeling angry, find a way to delay saying something to your child that you—or more importantly she—will regret afterwards. For example: Count

to ten, take a walk, turn on the radio or change the subject. Jacqueline, one of the parents in my Parents Advisory Group who specializes in imagery work shared a brief and effective breathing technique that can really work to calm you down: The focus during this exercise is on the *exhalation*. Begin by breathing normally. When you are ready, take a long slow exhalation followed by a brief inhalation. Begin a count of three cycles of breath with the exhalation; then, take another short, quick breath in, then count two with your second full, long exhalation; take a second quick breath in and then exhale fully for a third and final time, concentrating and relaxing. Remember, once you have said something that might be hurtful, you can never take it back, so be cautious about what you say in anger.

STEP THREE: Instead of saying something angry, change your words into something positive and affirming. You'd be amazed at the difference. Below are some examples. I'm sure you can think of plenty more that will work just as well, or even better for you and your child:

Instead of: You're so lazy, you never do any exercise!

Try: *I'd love some company on my walk today.*

Instead of: You ate all those cookies—no wonder you can't lose weight!

Try: *I see you really enjoy these cookies—I bet it would help you if I put them in portion sized baggies for you.*

Instead of: You look fat in that shirt.

Try: *That's not one of my favorite choices for you, but why don't you look in the mirror and decide for yourself how you feel in this shirt.*

STEP FOUR: You need to do your best to truly reduce or eliminate your anger, rather than merely repressing it. Repressed anger might become misdirected and targeted at another aspect of your child's life. You could then find yourself overreacting angrily to your child about something unrelated to her weight, such as school work or a messy room.

Guilt Can Really Get You

In my experience most parental guilt is misplaced. Parents expend *far too much* wasted energy feeling guilty about important life choices, such as working, how much time they spend with their kids, how much money they spend on their kids, even about getting divorced when necessary. Children suffer much more from the guilt-driven impulses parents give in to because their kids are nagging, than they suffer from well-thought out decisions made in the interest of raising emotionally healthy and well-behaved children.

Guilt is a common parental feeling! Parents feel guilty about many, many things. It comes from the *perception*—regardless of whether it is accurate—that you have done something to harm your child. How many of the following have YOU felt guilty about?

- I work too much

- I don't work at all

- I yell too much

- I'm divorced

- I travel too much without my child

- I don't spend enough time with my child

- I argue too much with my partner in front of my child

- I'm financially limited so my child doesn't get everything he needs/wants

- My child has a chronic medical illness/condition or psychological/learning issue and I feel either genetically responsible or just plain guilty that my child, rather than I got stuck dealing with this bad luck

- I feel guilty because_____(FILL IN YOUR OWN BLANK)

Parental guilt is a very powerful and stressful emotion, which, if you have experienced it, you will know, causes you to feel terribly sorry for your child, thinking that she must suffer with whatever the particular issue is that you are feeling guilty about—whether it is you working too much, getting divorced, not having enough money or_____(FILL IN THE BLANK).

The problem with feeling sorry for your child is that it makes it difficult for you to say "No!" to things, because you don't want to deprive a child that you feel is already deprived—right?

You're probably already seeing that this has a lot to do with your overweight child. When it comes to food and eating, *parental guilt* is a big factor in kids becoming and staying overweight. This is because food is one of the most difficult things to which parents have a hard time saying "NO!" Do any of the following sound similar to your family? If they do, perhaps you're struggling with parent guilt.

- When you come home from work it may be tough to say NO to a child who wants a donut because the NO might result in tears or anger. You'd rather say yes and have a calm couple of hours than have your precious time with your child ruined with a tantrum—you feel bad enough that you work so late.

- As a noncustodial parent you don't get that much time with your kids—why shouldn't they eat whatever they want when they're with you.

- Although money is tight, candy, ice cream, and chips are little money compared to the big ticket items, so it's easy to say "yes" to those a lot because you feel guilty about how often you have to say "NO" to the more expensive things.

- You know you have a short temper so you make up for it by buying your kids the junk food they always request.

- Your child has a learning disability and really struggles in school. You don't have the heart to say "No" when he asks for more food or extra snacks—even though you realize your child had a weight issue.

- You've had a death in your family and you feel sorry for your child—how can you deprive her of anything else.

Get Rid of Guilt

Guilt is not an easy feeling to reduce. But it can be done and it is well worth working at it. Allowing your child to overeat and eat too much of the wrong foods because you feel too guilty to set limits is clearly not good for your child's physical health, nor is it good for your relationship with your child. The following two steps will help you to get your guilt in check and your child's health on track!

STEP ONE: Take stock of the issues that cause you guilt and write them down. Review your list once a week or so, to see if it changes.

STEP TWO: Think about alternative ways to help you alleviate your guilt about your child's predicament that *do not involve food.* Write your alternatives down as well and keep your list with you so that you can refer to it whenever you get the urge to use food as a guilt pacifier.

It's a great idea to reread your list once a week or so to make sure that it doesn't need to be edited as you subtract issues you've mastered or add others you may think of. One of the parents in my Parents Advisory Group keeps a copy in her wallet and looks at it during spare moments—like when she's waiting for the train. She says it is helping her to become a more mindful parent.

Below are some examples to get you thinking. I'm confident you'll be able to think of your own as well:

- Instead of bringing home donuts when you've been working late, spend some time talking to your child or playing a game. You may not be happy that you had to work late, and your child may be angry with you, but it is healthy for your child to express this feeling to you, rather than for you to try and squash the feeling with food. This is an excellent example of how the food–mood connection can be effectively changed so that food isn't used to manage feelings.

- If you lose it in the department store when your kids hide in the clothing racks. Instead of assuaging your guilt with ice cream sundaes, apologize genuinely for embarrassing them in public. Nothing more is necessary. Addressing and validating your child's feelings are critical. Modeling healthy emotional behavior by showing your child you are capable of apologizing are of equal importance. Giving your child ice cream does nothing to further enhance your emotional commitment to your child in this or any situation. In fact, it could actually dilute the full impact of the interaction.

- When your child constantly asks for stuff even though you can't afford it, rather than giving her junk food just so you feel like you're giving *something*, start putting away all those coins and dollars that you might have spent on candy, chips, and soda—a piggy bank will do. You can even carry the bank with you, so your child can see the money going into the bank, rather than into her tummy! Before long you'll have enough money to get something that your child really wants—and maybe she will have slimmed down a bit too!

- When the twinge of divorce guilt makes you want to give your child everything under the sun, including all the junk food he wants, instead, spend a day or two before your time together planning a really great, physically active and busy visit that focuses on lots of movement (biking, skating, ball, swimming, hiking, etc.) and less on food. Being a good divorced parent is only partly about how much time you spend with your child. The other part is what you do with that time. Really great parenting (divorced or not) is about making the effort to do not what is easiest, but what is in the best interest of your child's emotional and physical health! Parents that are not divorced also may need to plan physically active days in advance to make sure that they take place—this is especially true for weekends and vacations.

The Frustration Factor

Frustration with your child is sometimes enough to make you throw up your hands and simply give up! We've all done it, haven't we? After what seems like the fiftieth time saying "No!" to candy, a second or third helping of something or to a can of soda you just can't take it anymore so you say "Yes." Or when your "No" results in a temper tantrum, screaming fit or other unpleasant reaction, perhaps you say "Yes" just to end the behavior.

But, if this is happening several times a week or even several times a day, there's a good chance that it is at least part of the reason your child is overweight. There are two very good reasons that *now* is an excellent time to stop using food as a way to manage your frustration with your child's behavior.

I. Your child's physical and emotional health are both at risk when too much food and junk food is eaten—no matter what the reason.

2. Learning to cope with frustration is one *of the most important* **life skills** you will ever teach your child! When you give in to a temper tantrum, nag or crying spell, you send your child the message that

he never needs to experience frustration, as long as he persists long enough being unpleasant, rude or hostile. This is not a message that will get your child very far in real life.

Fixing Your Frustration

If you are experiencing ongoing frustration with your child (or children's) behavior and feel that you're constantly giving in to nagging and temper tantrums or that you can't seem to keep control, it is likely that your frustration represents a larger issue than just giving in to food. So, in order for you to accomplish your goals of reducing your frustration it will mean that you will need to learn how to manage your child or children without feeling that you need to give in to their negative behavior. To do this I strongly recommend the following suggestions—they will make being a parent much more rewarding because if you really follow them, your children will become much better behaved:

1. If you are following a plan (like *Kids-Only Weight Loss Guide*) to help your child lose weight or eat more healthily then when you make a rule or decision not to give your child another helping or a junk food snack, you **must** stick to it. Don't give in to temper tantrums, crying fits or any other form of nagging or abusive behavior trying to convince you to change your mind. By not giving in to these behaviors you teach your child that they are not effective. Soon, you will find that your child will not try them on you nearly as often.

2. Before going to eat in a restaurant, give your child the options that he may choose from on the menu (see Chapter Seven for suggestions in each restaurant category). This includes reminding your child that soda is not an option, and also which (if any) choices you approve of for dessert. This way, when you get into the restaurant and look at the menu together, there will be a greatly reduced chance of stress and fighting. It is important to stick to the options you negotiated, no matter how much your child tries to convince you otherwise, once he's had a chance to examine the menu.

REMEMBER: Learning Frustration Tolerance is a critical life skill for your child.

3. Don't promise, threaten or suggest doing anything to or with your child—either positive or negative—that you absolutely, positively are not willing to follow-through with (i.e., don't threaten a punishment and then retract it because it's not convenient for you). This rule applies to food related issues and all other issues as well. It will help your child learn that when you say something you really mean it!

4. Don't embarrass your child in public by yelling, demeaning or reprimanding her—if you want your child to respect you, you must also respect your child.

5. Before you do anything or go anywhere, make the rules and consequences clear. Then **follow through**.

❖ ❖ ❖ ❖ ❖

CONGRATULATIONS!!! You have made it through a very important chapter. I am sure that you are doing great. If you'd like to check in with me and tell me how you're doing so far, you can reach me at DrSusan@ kidsonlyweightloss.com.

The Real Road to a Healthier Child

Now that we've taken a careful look at the many different factors that could be contributing to your child being overweight, I am sure you are beginning to have a much better idea about what you can be doing to help your child become healthier. In fact, I'm sure you're already making many of the changes we've discussed in the first five chapters!

Here in Chapter Six, we'll get to the nuts and bolts of healthy eating! You'll discover that feeding your child healthily is really quite simple and that you will be able to learn how to do it with little trouble.

But before we begin to discuss the things you *should* be doing to help your child lose weight and become healthier, let's take a quick look at the approaches to eating that *don't* work well with children and some that might even be dangerous.

Dieting Dangers

In Chapter One, we talked a little about the issue of dieting, but it's such an important subject that it bears further discussion.

It can be tempting to place a child on a formal diet—perhaps one of the diets that you have tried, or that you are currently finding successful. But diets created for adults are not safe for a child's, or even a teen's, body. Children and teens require different types and amounts of foods than adults. If children don't get enough protein, fat, carbohydrates, vitamins, minerals, fiber, and water that their bodies require, they may not grow up healthily and their thinking, memory, energy, and strength could be negatively affected. In other words, *diets that are formulated for adults are **not** meant for the bodies of children or teens.*

Fat-Free and Nonfat Foods

Low fat foods are very useful and should definitely be included on your shopping list when you are helping your child to lose weight and become healthier. We'll talk more about this later in this chapter.

Even fat-free or nonfat foods can be a part of your child's life. But, it is very important not to make fat-free foods the *only* foods your child eats. Foods that contain no fat do not usually taste as filling or as satisfying as the same foods with fat. Take cookies for example...the fat-free kind just don't taste as good, do they? Guess what, they don't really have that many fewer calories either! Your child (or you) may actually consume more calories eating fat-free cookies, trying to satisfy your cookie urge than you would by eating one or two real, full-fat cookies. In addition, since the human body does not manufacture its own essential fatty acids, we must get them from our diet. Essential fatty acids promote healthy skin and hair, support proper thyroid function and adrenal activity, and bolster immunity, brain activity, normal growth process, and energy. So, including them in your child's regular diet is important. While it's better to get fats from healthier foods (which you'll learn about later in the chapter) a full-fat treat once in a while is okay too.

As you read the rest of this chapter, you will learn all about how to make sure your child eats healthily without feeling deprived. Balancing health and delicious taste is a part of that!!

Artificial Sweeteners

The food industry uses many different low or no-calorie artificial sweeteners instead of sugar to sweeten food and drinks. These include saccharin (Sweet'n Low), aspartame (Equal, NutraSweet), sucralose (Splenda), and acesulfame potassium (Sunnett).

Artificial sweeteners certainly have an important place in the lives of those trying to lose weight and particularly for people with diabetes. However scientific controversy does exist as to whether artificial sweeteners are safe. Saccharin in particular has been labeled with cautions that it has been shown to cause cancer in lab animals. Since the other sweeteners are much newer, the jury is still out as to their long-term safety for people.

Each parent needs to make a personal decision as to the use of artificial sweeteners and many different philosophies exist, even amongst friends—I've had many debates with mine! But, since we really can't be absolutely sure how safe these are for children, it's safe to say that artificial sweeteners shouldn't be relied upon in large amounts as part of your child's healthy eating program, nor should you count on them as typical substitute for other higher-calorie snacks. As you will learn in this chapter (and will teach your child), eating the right size portions of healthy foods is going to be the best way to better health. Artificial sweeteners may let your child eat a few more bites of food, but they won't help your child make the life changes that will make the real difference!

Beverages seem to spark the greatest debate about allowing children artificial sweeteners. I would suggest that water (flavored with fruit slices if you like) or flavored seltzer should always be the first drink you offer your child. But if sugar-sweetened sodas, juices, and drinks have been a large part of your child's life until you began this new healthier lifestyle, it is okay to substitute diet beverages in moderation (about one cup a day) to ease the transition.

Drastic Calorie Restrictions

The way to lose weight—everyone knows—is to *eat fewer calories*—right!! It can therefore be tempting to jumpstart your child's weight loss by really slashing the number of calories he eats each day.

Actually, this is a surefire way to making sure that your child *doesn't* succeed at losing weight. Kids need to eat enough calories each day in order to have energy for school, homework, sports, playing, thinking, sleeping, and growing. If they don't get these calories they will be cranky, tired, distracted, angry, sad, have difficulty thinking, and even have physical symptoms, such as headaches and stomachaches.

What's more, if one's body doesn't get enough calories consistently, their body will hold onto every single calorie that it gets since the metabolism slows down, and it then becomes even more difficult to lose weight. So, by not making sure your child is eating enough food, you might actually be making it harder for your child to lose weight!

In addition to these potential problems, being overly restricting places your child at risk for developing an eating disorder because he may begin to sneak food, eat secretly or binge eat (see Chapter Four, Pattern #2: Forbidden Foods, if you want to read more about this).

If you are concerned about how to reduce the number of calories that your child is eating then, as you read the rest of this chapter, pay close attention to the ways in which you can reduce calories without leaving your child feeling hungry or deprived.

Now that we have cleared up all the ways not to do it, we're ready to talk about the best, most effective, and healthiest way to help your child make the important eating changes that reflect the beginning of a lifetime of healthy eating.

There are three simple steps that you must take with your child down this path toward healthy eating. I will show you the way and take the steps with you. These steps work together to make sure that your child is (a) eating healthily and (b) is not feeling deprived. *All* of these are critical in order for your child (and, of course, you) to experience long-term success. The three steps are:

STEP ONE: Help your child make healthier choices.

STEP TWO: Teach your child to eat smaller portions.

STEP THREE: Make sure your child eats enough and isn't deprived of foods she loves.

I will discuss each of these in detail so you learn how to use them in your child's life and teach them to your child so he can learn to use them independently. You can work on the steps together or one at a time. Be patient with yourself. Remember, your child didn't gain weight overnight, so learning healthier ways will likely take months or even years. As long as you keep working at it, you and your child have every reason to feel proud of yourselves! Once you can consistently apply these three ideas to your child's life, then you and your child (and maybe your whole family) will really begin to notice big, wonderful changes!

STEP ONE: Make Healthier Food Choices

Many children are overweight because they or their parents don't choose healthy foods often enough. Often this is because you aren't sure how to determine if a food is healthy. So, I'm going to make it simple for you! There are four categories to consider when deciding the health value of a food. I've called these categories the **Main Menu, Consume with Care, Largely Liquid,** and **Sweets and Treats**. Each category should be included in your child's life in a different way.

The Main Menu

The foods in this category give your child's body the energy (calories) it needs to function and grow. These foods fall into many groups, providing your child's body with a variety of nutrients (protein, carbohydrates, fat, fiber, vitamins, and minerals) it requires, without overdoing the fat or calories.

Dr. Judy Marshel (you can learn more about her in Appendix Two), a fantastic dietician who specializes in children and teens' nutrition, explained the details of all the information we need to know about **Main Menu** foods.

Protein

It is very important for children to eat protein foods throughout the day when they are trying to lose weight (or *stretch out* as they grow in height without gaining much weight) because protein is the food that is **best** at keeping a child (or anyone) from feeling hungry. Foods containing protein include poultry (without skin), lean meat, fish, dairy, beans, eggs, soy, lentils, and nuts). If I haven't convinced you yet of the importance of protein, take a look at all that it does for your child's body:

- Has vitamins and minerals necessary for bone growth

- Builds, repairs, and maintains muscles and all other tissues

- Helps grow and maintain bones, teeth, hair, and fingernails

- Transports nutrients in and out of cells

- Helps maintain a healthy immune system

- Is a major part of all hormones and digestive enzymes

NOTE: Healthy proteins can be disguised in a way that makes them less healthy. For example, healthy chicken or fish become less healthy when you deep-fry them in cooking oil, adding lots of extra fat, or when you decide to eat the skin on the chicken, rather than taking it off. Later in this chapter and in Chapter Seven, we'll discuss this in detail.

Carbohydrates and Fiber

Carbohydrates (sometimes known as carbs) are a somewhat more complicated category than proteins because some carbohydrates are healthy, while others are less healthy. For example, sugar (and any food very high in sugar) is a type of carbohydrate that contains very few nutrients and is therefore not very healthy. I will discuss more about sugar in the **Sweets and Treats** section.

Foods like whole grain pasta, brown rice, and whole grain bread are nutritious carbohydrates, which provide your child's body with fuel for energy throughout the day. Look for the words *whole grain* foods (it should say so *on the label*) because they have more vitamins, minerals, and fiber (which helps your child feel full and aids digestion) than other similar foods.

Fruits and vegetables are also carbohydrates that give your child fiber as well as energy. In addition, they are a great source of vitamins and minerals. Frozen fruits and vegetables are just as good fresh, so keep plenty on hand. In fact, sometimes frozen fruits and vegetables are even more nutritious than fresh. This is because fresh produce begins to lose its nutritional value as soon as it is picked. On the other hand, frozen vegetables and fruits are flash frozen at the peak of their freshness so that all the nutrients are frozen right in, ready for your child to eat, so these are likely to be fresher than produce that has been waiting to be purchased at the market for more than a couple of days. On the other hand, *fruit juice is not a good substitute for fresh fruit* and, in fact, like sugary soda, too much fruit juice is one of the biggest causes of weight gain in children.

One of the best ways to feed your child healthy fruits and veggies is to camouflage them! For example, pizza sauce has the benefit of tomatoes, onions, and garlic. On the other hand, like proteins, it's also possible to disguise healthy fruits and vegetables so that they become *less* healthy. For example when you deep fry vegetables tempura-style, so much extra fat is added that the benefit of eating a vegetable is lost.

Others carbohydrates are not as nutritious or high in fiber as fruit and vegetables, but not as devoid of nutritional value as **Sweets and Treats** either. These are foods such as crackers, white bread, white rice, many kids' breakfast cereals, and other carbohydrates that are low in protein and low in fiber. There is a place in every child (and adult's) life for these foods, but they belong in the **Consume with Care** section.

Some examples of these carbohydrates are white bread, white rice, refined pasta, bagels, donuts, and many breakfast cereals. Dr. Dhuper explained that these foods are refined starch that is made up of many small molecules of glucose (sugar). They get digested very quickly and lead to a sudden spike in blood sugar. This then leads to your child's body producing extra of a hormone called insulin, which is needed to try and digest the sugar, which *then* leads to a rapid decline in the blood sugar, creating hunger and cravings for more starchy, sugary foods. This could become a vicious cycle and lead to your child overeating. Believe it or not even potatoes fall into this category and unless your child is extremely active during the day, all the extra starch can be converted into fat and stored. Dr. Dhuper says to remember, if you don't burn it off, you store it. When we get to Chapter Nine, we'll talk about burning it off!

Healthy Fats

Although you may have been brainwashed to think otherwise by years of dieting and fashion magazines, believe it or not everybody needs to eat fat. But this is especially true for children! In addition, as we have discussed, foods that contain fat are more satisfying to our child's taste buds and stomach than fat-free foods.

But, admittedly, incorporating fat into your child's daily eating can be tricky, because some types of fat aren't as healthy as other types. For example, the kind of fat found in cookies, cake, red meat, butter, mayonnaise, whole milk or other full-fat dairy products is not as beneficial as the types of fats found in fatty fish (e.g., salmon, mackerel, bluefish, sardines), nuts, seeds, and some vegetables, like avocados and olives, as well as canola oil and olive oil. These fats are important because they:

- Keep skin and hair healthy

- Help heal wounds

- Maintain a healthy nervous system

- Make hormones

- Slow down digestion and the emptying of food out of your stomach, so you feel satisfied longer. This is why, if you feed your child only no-fat or very low-fat foods he will feel hungry all the time and will eat more often, which could result in your child actually eating more calories than if you feed your child some fat.

You need to become a food label reader and watch out for and avoid foods that have trans fats and partially hydrogenated oils. These are not only unhealthy, Dr. Dhuper notes they are dangerous for one's heart. It is also important to avoid unhealthy saturated fats. Healthy fats to look for and include in your child's diet are those that are polyunsaturated and monounsaturated fats. These are heart healthy and can be used liberally when cooking. The key is to make sure your child eats mostly healthy fats, and then balance them with enough protein and healthy carbohydrates. Keep reading and we'll discuss how to do this.

Consume with Care

The foods in this group contain some healthy nutrients, but may also be high in calories, fat or both. Regular pizza is a good example of a **Consume with Care** food. The sauce is made of healthy vegetables and cheese has some protein and calcium. But mozzarella cheese also has the less healthy kind of fat. These foods should definitely be a part of your child's new eating plan, but they should be balanced with foods that contain healthy fats. Other examples of **Consume with Care** foods are:

- Chicken with skin and fatty red meat (hot dogs, nonlean beef or pork, lamb (these have protein, but lots of fat)

- Full-fat (not low-fat or nonfat) dairy products (hard cheese, cottage cheese, yogurt, cream, sour cream), and peanut butter, all or which have protein but, *when eaten in excess*, a lot of fat

- Creamy pasta sauces (if your child eats *a lot* of sauce[s] she is eating a great deal of fat)

- Refined carbohydrates such as *non*whole grain crackers and bread, highly sweetened cereals, white rice, white pasta

Largely Liquid

The third category, **Largely Liquid**, consists of foods such a celery, lettuce, spinach, green peppers, cucumbers, and radishes, which are made mostly of water. Most have good nutritional value and lots of fiber, and all have very few calories. These should definitely be included in your child's new eating plan daily but, no matter how tempting it is to do so, you should never allow them to take the place of foods in the **Main Menu** or **Consume with Care** categories. Foods like this may be low in calories but they should be an addition, not a substitution.

Trying New Foods

For some parents getting a child to eat **Largely Liquid** (or any!) foods can be a challenge. But, since these are nutritious and can be an excellent substitute for higher calorie snacks, it is worth making the commitment to helping your child to learn to eat them. Research shows that when children's taste buds are exposed to a new food frequently, over a short period of time, they often grow to like it. So, here's a quick 3-step program that often works with almost any food if you stick to it!

1. If your child is old enough to understand, explain that you are going to be helping him learn how to eat new foods. Then, pick a food you want your child to learn to eat—start with one that is commonly eaten by kids (an older child will be more motivated if given their own choice).

2. For seven days in a row *at the beginning* of a meal give your child a tiny (less than the size of your smallest finger nail)

piece of the new food to try. You may increase the size of the piece only if your child is willing to eat more, or—even better—enjoys it. Each time give your child lots of praise, hugs, and kisses for doing great trying, even if she is somewhat resistant. If your child simply can't stand the food, is gagging, throwing up or otherwise disgusted, try another food starting the next night—perhaps with a different texture. Remember to also teach by example. Eat each of the new foods along with your child at each meal. You can even ask your child for hugs, kisses, and praise when you try something new!

3. On day eight, do an assessment. Perhaps by now your child is already eating larger amounts of the food. Otherwise, if your child is willing to try a *slightly* larger piece at this point, then repeat step two again patiently. Don't rush—the two or three (or more) weeks investment will be worth it, because in the end, your child's healthy food repertoire will be increased. Continue to compliment and praise your child for trying and for succeeding. Don't worry about foods that your child simply can't stand. There are so many others to try.

Once you have mastered one food, you can move onto others—there is no limit. Have fun! Some parents make up colorful, fun charts that help them and their kids to keep track of the foods they have tried. Let me know what works for you by emailing me at DrSusan@kidsonlyweightloss.com.

Sweets and Treats

The last category, **Sweets and Treats** includes foods that taste good, but provide little or no nutritional value for your child's body. In addition, unlike the **Largely Liquid** foods, these are not low or no calorie. You may hear these types of foods referred to as "empty calories" because they don't give one's body nutrients, but they do have a significant number of extra calories from sugar and fat. These are the foods that children love, and usually eat too much of and too often. These are the foods that they beg us for in the supermarket, tantrum for at night, and plead for after school. Along with **Consume with Care** foods, too many **Sweets and Treats** can cause your child to become overweight.

Examples of foods in this category are cookies, potato and tortilla chips, ice cream, cake, candy, pie, fried treats (like french fries and donuts), soda, and sports drinks. I place fruit juices and drinks into this category as well, even though they are technically made of fruit. This is because they are mostly made up of sugar—even if it is naturally produced sugar (as in pure apple juice). Dr. Marshel says that up to one cup of 100 percent fruit juice a day is fine, but more than that is too much sugar and calories.

Despite the fact that they are not nutritious, you *should not* stop allowing your child to eat these foods completely. Having read the first part of this book, you probably understand by now that this is because it will cause her to feel deprived, frustrated, and resentful. There is a place in your child's life for every type of food, including "junk-food." When you read the next two steps, you will learn how to incorporate these foods into your child's new eating plan.

Sensational Substitutions (Part 1)

One of the concerns I hear most often from parents is that they are afraid to introduce healthy food into their child's life because they think their child will hate it and refuse to eat it.

Peggy, the mother of Jackie (7) and Steven (10) shared her feelings: "my husband and I can't get our kids to eat food like salad, salmon, and brown rice! They'll go crazy if I try to bring healthy food into the house, I'll have a mutiny on my hands!"

Peggy doesn't realize that children can eat healthily without needing to give up the yummy "kid" food that they love. One of the great things I am about to show you about how to teach your child more healthily is that there are many different ways that you can take the foods that your child likes and **make** them healthy.

Just because a food isn't in the **Main Menu** category doesn't mean that it can't become healthier. In fact, some of your child's favorite foods can be changed and substitutes can be made to make them more nutritious and sometimes push them right onto your child's **Main Menu**. Below are some examples:

- **French Toast:** For the batter, use fat-free or low-fat milk instead of whole milk, and use 100 percent whole wheat instead of white bread. Give your child just a little syrup, for flavor.

- **Peanut butter and jelly sandwich:** Use all natural peanut butter (read the label to make sure peanuts are the only ingredient), 100 percent whole wheat bread, and real fruit jam instead of jelly.

- **Tuna salad sandwich:** Instead of regular mayonnaise, mix tuna with a bit of low-fat mayonnaise and add some lettuce and tomatoes (if your child will go for it). Don't forget the whole wheat bread!

- **Chicken nuggets:** There's not much you can do with these in a restaurant, but at home you can bake them instead of frying them. Just use a little oil spray on the pan and on the chicken so they don't dry out as they cook.

- **Breakfast cereal:** Mix your child's favorite sugary cereal with a low sugar cereal (e.g., Honey Nut Cheerios mixed with Total or Frosted Flakes mixed with bran flakes) and use low-fat instead of whole milk.

- **Hamburger:** Purchase *lean* ground meat or try ground chicken or turkey. Sneak some finely chopped onion, carrots or other veggies into the burger for added nutrition. My husband, Lewis' special burger recipe calls for onion soup powder mixed with ground turkey—it's delicious! Serve with veggies as a side dish instead of fries. Or serve the burger *without* the bun but *with* some fries (we'll discuss serving sizes in a few pages!)

- **Pizza:** As I mentioned, a slice of pizza is actually quite a well balanced meal for a child—it has protein, veggies, and carbs. If you special order your child's slice of pizza, asking for less cheese, you will cut down significantly on the amount of dairy fat. Pair this with seltzer or water, rather than soda. If you can convince your child to eat a salad (or even just pick on the veggies he likes), you've got a great meal! You can even sneak in a small Italian ice for dessert.

It is impossible for me to list every single successful Sensational Substitution because each child's taste is different. But you know your child. Now is the time for you to get creative, and to really start thinking about the ways you can change your child's favorites to make them healthier, without sacrificing too much of the flavor and the fun. Here are a couple of steps to jump start you:

1. Make a list of the meals and snacks your child eats regularly in your home every week. These are the foods for which it will be most important to find healthy substitutions that your child *really enjoys*.

2. Study the meals and snacks on your list, breaking each one down into individual ingredients. As you look at the ingredients, decide whether each falls into the **Main Menu, Consume with Care, Largely Liquid,** or **Sweets and Treats** category. Then, as I did in the examples above, look for a way to substitute a healthier ingredient for one that falls into the **Consume with Care** or **Sweets and Treats** group. In most cases you will be able to make a meal or snack much healthier without your child having to sacrifice taste. As with any new experience, you will get better and better at doing this the more you practice. Before long you will become an expert

at seeking out the most well-stocked stores with the healthiest foods and best, most sensational substitutions. And when you do, don't forget to email them to me at sensationalsubstitutions@kids onlyweightloss.com.

3. If you find a food for which there is simply no healthier substitution, read Step #2: Teach your child to eat smaller portions and Step #3: Make sure your child isn't deprived of foods she loves.

STEP TWO: Teach Your Child to Eat Smaller Portions

Everywhere we go we are encouraged to buy and eat larger amounts of food. Restaurants and food markets compete for customers by promising more food at lower prices than the next one is selling. It tempts us every time, doesn't it? Unfortunately, the "bigger is better," "more for your money" way of life is contributing to adults, children, and teenagers becoming fatter now than they have ever been in history. For some reason, we don't want to resist a deal, with our bodies paying the price.

I have a confession...I once bought a box of cookies so large that it should have taken my whole family (there are five of us) six months to finish it (I couldn't resist, it was on sale!). But, since the cookies were right there, and since there were so many, we all ate cookies everyday. The box was empty in two weeks. I know I'm not alone. Have you ever ordered the extra-large fries because they're only thirty cents more than the small? Come home with eight boxes of cheese crackers because there was a two-for-one sale? Eaten (or allowed your child to eat) six pieces of garlic bread because it's free on the table, and then a huge plate of pasta that you ordered? Bought a super size candy bar for your child because you get 25 percent more free? Or let everyone gorge themselves on popcorn and soda before the movie even begins and then run back out to get your free refill on your jumbo popcorn and free soda? If you answered "yes" to any of the above "good deals" you'll find this section very interesting.

Since we are surrounded by huge amounts of food, supersized everything and supposedly great value for our money, it's easy to lose sight of how much your child is actually eating compared to how much her body actually really needs. It is also very easy to lose sight of what a healthy serving size actually looks like.

Dr. Marshel, our wonderful dietician, gave me some quick and easy tips to help us figure out what a healthy serving size looks like for many of your child's favorite foods.

- A serving of cooked pasta, rice, fruit, cereal, or cooked vegetables is equal to an adult or teen's closed fist or a child's slightly open fist or a baseball (about one cup).

- A serving of a baked potato is the size of a computer mouse. If you only get large potatoes, give your child half a potato.

- A serving of cold cereal is two handfuls (about a cup). Teach your child to use the same size bowl each morning. Use a measuring cup once or twice to see where the cereal should measure up to in the bowl. Then your child will be able to pour a healthy portion of cereal each morning, independently without measuring. You may need to check in once in a while and get out the measuring cup to make sure the portion isn't creeping up again over time. Instead of a second bowl of cereal, offer a piece of fruit.

- A serving of a bagel is the size of a makeup compact or a hockey puck (wow, Dr. Marshel that is small!). Many bagels are two or three times this size. Only purchase mini-bagels for your child or offer half the bagel instead with a piece of fruit.

- A serving of butter, margarine, cream cheese or mayonnaise is equal to the tip of your thumb to the first joint (about one tablespoon). Keep this in mind when you're making sandwiches for your child.

- A serving of peanut butter is the size of a golf or ping pong ball (about two tablespoons).

- A serving of meat, chicken, turkey or fish is about the size of the palm of a woman's palm, a bar of soap, or a deck of cards. This is the amount to give your child at a meal as a first helping along with a serving of vegetables and a serving of carbohydrates (don't forget serving sizes for carbs too!). If your child wants a second helping, remember to wait fifteen minutes and then offer a piece of fruit.

- A serving of a muffin (corn, bran, chocolate chip, etc.) is the size of two large eggs or a softball. It is *not* the size of one of those huge bakery muffins that many people give their kids, thinking it's a healthy snack.

- A serving of cheese is one string cheese, or it's the size of an adult's index finger, or the shape of an index card (American or sliced cheese).

- A serving of a waffle or pancake is equal to a CD (in circumference, not depth).

- A serving of a burger is the size of a palm of a woman's hand.

- A serving of french fries is ten fries (yes, that's TEN!).

- A serving of pizza is one slice (an 1/8 of a pie).

- A serving of chips or pretzels is about fourteen.

- A serving of ice cream or frozen yogurt is one scoop (about ½ a cup).

- A serving of juice or soda is one cup.

- A serving of lite popcorn is about three cups.

If you're not sure what a serving size is for a particular food, you can usually look at the "Nutrition Facts" label on the back of the package. The first item is always Serving Size.

Sneaky Serving Sizes

There is a big problem with some food labels that it is important to be aware of as both a parent and as a consumer. In order to encourage sales, some food manufacturers label their products in a way that makes them look as if they are low-calorie or low-fat, when they really aren't. They do this by *making the serving sizes unreasonably small.* For example, many kids love Snapple and parents buy it, thinking it's a healthier alternative to soda. But, if you look at the 8 oz bottle of Snapple carefully it tells you that it contains *two* servings. This means you have to double the calories and sugar your child is consuming. Calorie for calorie, sugar gram for sugar gram, Snapple is no healthier than soda.

But, I'm not just picking on Snapple. I've seen the same thing on labels of *individual* size potato chips (a bag contains two servings—could you expect your child to eat half a small bag of chips? Of course not!) and even on a package of muffins—one small muffin was two servings! As an experiment, take a walk in the supermarket and carefully read the labels on your child's favorite snack foods. I'm sure you'll also be surprised as to how many "single serving" foods actually contain more than one serving according to the package.

For your child's health, it's important for you to be an educated consumer. Just as you are now teaching your child about the impact the media can have on eating habits and body image, so too must you teach your child how the food industry packages products to look attractive and encourage purchasing, rather than packaging them in a way that is honest and forthright with consumers.

STEP THREE: Make Sure Your Child Eats Enough and Isn't Deprived of Foods He Loves

Steps two and three may seem contradictory at first—how can you limit portions and also make sure your child eats enough and is not deprived? But actually they complement each other very well. Eating smaller portions does not mean your child should be hungry, nor does it mean your child should feel deprived of foods (often **sweets and treats**) that he loves to eat.

Making sure your child doesn't feel hungry is one of your most important goals! Accomplishing it will ensure that your child is able to eat smaller portions and feel satisfied. Most importantly, it means that your child will continue to be able to do so over *not only days and weeks, but months and years.*

Create Your Main Menu Shopping List

In order to make sure your child doesn't feel hungry it is very important that you feed your child foods that are *filling* and *satisfying*. If you take a quick look back at Step One, you will see that protein foods help to keep your child feeling satisfied. This is because they do not cause your blood sugar to jump up and down. Simple carbohydrates (like sugars) get used up very quickly by one's body so your child will likely feel hungry again sooner. Also, excellent at serving this purpose are whole grain carbohydrates and fresh fruits and vegetables. For the most part—**Main Menu** foods are the ones that you need to keep really well stocked!

The best way to keep your fridge and pantry full of these healthy foods is to figure out which ones your child likes the best. This takes trial and error. For example, you may need to try different fruits and vegetables before you hit on a few that your child enjoys (and don't forget the **trying new foods** technique). In our house, broccoli is a staple—my three kids eat it almost *every single night* because they all enjoy it and it's really healthy. Apples, eggs, and grilled chicken are other regular healthy foods in our home. We go through about two dozen apples a week, at least two dozen eggs (some only enjoy the whites, some the whole egg), and at least eight pounds of chicken (we eat it hot, cold, and as sandwiches!).

As you find healthy foods that your child really enjoys add them to your shopping list and make sure that you have them always available as the *first foods you offer your hungry child*. And when you offer these foods, always remember Step Two—portion sizes.

Healthy Snacks Are Also Important

As you are stocking your new, healthier pantry and fridge with snack foods, you should apply the same rules as you do for meals—do your best to look for foods that are in the **Main Menu, Consume with Care**, or **Largely Liquid** categories. In addition, it is particularly important to be as creative as possible with **Sensational Substitutions** when looking for snack foods.

While you always want to make healthy snacks your first choice, this is also the time when you will want to allow children to eat some foods in the **Sweets and Treats** category as long as you teach them about portion control (snack size baggies for you to make your own portions, or pre-packaged low calorie snacks are excellent for this purpose). This is because overweight children are sensitive about wanting to feel just like everyone else when it comes to snacking. *Being completely denied the snack foods your child enjoys will be one of the main reasons a healthy eating plan could fail, because your child will become extremely resistant and angry.*

In order to dramatically improve the likelihood of success I strongly suggest that you include at least one (and sometimes two) *portion controlled* (read the label to see what a portion is for the snack your child chooses) **Sweets and Treats** snack each day. Allow your child to choose when she would like the snack. Most children want it in their lunch box, after school, when having a playdate, or after dinner. On the other hand, including more than two **Sweets and Treats** foods will undermine your child's healthy eating, even if it is in smaller portions than she has been used to. For this reason, all other snacks should come from the **Main Menu, Consume with Care,** or **Largely Liquid** groups.

Sensational Substitutions (Part II)

Helping your child feel satisfied with snacks, while making sure that they are as healthy as possible takes some creativity as well as decision making! Sometimes your child will only be satisfied with exactly what he wants and no substitute will do. In this case, it's all about portion size—a couple of cookies are fine, a whole sleeve of them isn't. In fact, choosing the low-fat or fat-free substitute may not even be a better option because although it may be less fat, it may be about the same number of calories and much less tasty, leaving your child *far* less satisfied and still craving the original cookie. This defeats the purpose.

But in many cases, your child will be satisfied with a healthier substitution, if you can just find the right one. Take chocolate, for example. Your child may want a large candy bar, but would be satisfied with a bowl of chocolate cereal and low-fat milk, a small chocolate frozen yogurt, a couple of Tootsie Roll mini's, or a handful of M&M's. Dr. Dhuper suggests a couple of Dove Dark Chocolate Miniatures as a treat. Dark chocolate is packed with antioxidants, which are cancer fighting and heart protective. Better yet, mix them with warm low-fat or fat-free milk and serve them as hot chocolate (it's healthier and more fun than the powdered varieties).

Below are a few more ideas that might work to get you and your child through some **Sweets and Treats** tough times. With each suggestion, keep portions in mind. Don't forget to email your great ideas for sensational substitutions at sensationalsubstitutions@kidsonlyweightloss.com.

- If your child is craving the salty crunch of potato chips, instead try pretzels, salted air-popped popcorn or a couple of rice cakes. Put a serving in a bowl or on a plate and put the rest away.

- When your child wants a glazed donut, maybe a donut hole, a handful of jelly beans, a lollipop or a cup of caramel popcorn would be satisfying.

- You're being nagged for a large peanut butter chunk ice cream cone. Instead offer a small peanut butter frozen yogurt or sorbet or simply order a smaller scoop of ice cream.

What About Picky Eaters?

One of the most common concerns I hear from parents is echoed in this concern voiced by Lydia, mother to Donielle (8):

> **"**All Donielle will eat is pasta, grilled cheese, chicken nuggets, and, of course, junk food. The only fruit she'll touch is bananas and once in a while, she'll eat an apple if we cut it up for her. It's really difficult because the doctor has told us she's very overweight, but we don't know how to get her to eat the right foods without a real problem.**"**

It's very difficult when you have a very picky eater—but not impossible! It just takes a bit more patience. In Donielle's case, Lydia and Donielle's dad, Timothy, need to make a concerted effort to really capitalize on the healthy foods that Donielle will eat. For example, she will eat cut up apples. While this is a bit of extra work, they should expect to cut up apples every day for her, and Donielle needs to be told to expect to eat an apple at least once a day. In addition, they should immediately start trying new foods with Donielle, one at a time.

Chicken nuggets are a good candidate for a Sensational Substitution. They can be made at home using bread crumbs and they can be baked using a little oil spray, instead of deep frying them. Grilled cheese can be made with less cheese and so can pizza. That's just the start! Following the suggestions in the rest of this chapter, I'm sure there are other healthy foods and snacks that Donielle could grow to enjoy—given patience and time. I'm sure the same is true for your picky eater too.

"I'm Still Hungry"

Now that you know how to shop for healthier foods and serve them in carefully prepared portions, what does it mean and what do you do when your child finishes a meal and automatically asks for seconds.

There are two possible reasons for this:

1. Your child really is still hungry or

2. This is an automatic request that has little or nothing to do with hunger.

In either case, take the following steps at every meal to ensure that your child is not hungry. This will also alleviate any anxiety you may feel as well that you are allowing your child to leave the table hungry. When your child finishes a meal and says "I'm still hungry"

STEP ONE: Offer a second helping of vegetables or salad, or a piece of fruit.

STEP TWO: Remind your child that it takes at least fifteen minutes for his brain to register what is in his stomach. Tell him that he needs to wait the fifteen minutes before having anymore food.

STEP THREE: If he truly is still hungry he will come back in fifteen minutes for more food. At this point you can give him a small second helping of dinner, or another piece of fruit. If, after fifteen minutes he isn't hungry, hopefully he will have moved on to another activity. Even if he does request more food, by not having given in to his immediate request, you are teaching him to wait and to think about what his body is telling him.

A Note for Vegetarian (and Semi-Vegetarian) Families

For many different reasons, parents may choose to raise their children as vegetarians (not eating meat, fish or poultry); as lacto-ovo vegetarians (who include dairy product and eggs in their diets); as vegans (who avoid all animal products); or a personal variation of any of the above. In other cases, children decide that they don't *like* meat and choose to eat as vegetarians even though the rest of their family may not be. Finally, some parents decide that gradually (or at times abruptly) converting their child, or family, to a vegetarian lifestyle might be a good way to try and lose weight.

Actually, omitting animal based foods from your child's regular diet can be very healthy. In fact studies have shown that people who rely more on a vegetable-based diet are less likely to become very overweight than those who consume a great deal of meat—don't let anyone tell you otherwise! But doing so simply as a means to lose weight, can backfire if you do it abruptly without knowledge or planning. Your child could become confused or resentful. So, if your child is not vegetarian already, a better idea would be to gradually introduce vegetarian foods, and make the changeover a little at a time as you learn more about how to do so healthily. This section will provide you with a brief jumping off point. There is a lot more to learn. Appendix Three has further resources.

It is important to recognize that when a child doesn't eat animal based proteins (like meat, fish, poultry, and dairy) these need to be replaced by other healthy proteins. If not—since children are not always adventurous eaters—your children may begin to rely largely on familiar carbohydrates to feel satisfied. You'll remember from Step One that eating too many refined carbohydrates can lead to weight gain. In addition, the lack of variety in a bread, pasta, crackers, and dry cereal type of diet, could lead to your child becoming deficient in protein and other essential nutrients.

But, being a healthy vegetarian is definitely possible for all children. So, to give you some great ideas for beginning or keeping your vegetarian lifestyle while you help your child become healthier, I consulted with Dr. Reed Mangels (read more about her in Appendix Two), a registered dietician and Nutrition Advisor for the nonprofit *Vegetarian Resource Group*. She provided the most important information necessary to raise a healthy vegetarian child.

Dr. Mangels pointed out that eating healthily as a vegetarian may require a little extra thought and meal planning. This is because it can be a bit more challenging to make sure nutritional needs are fully met if your child doesn't eat the most available sources of protein—meat, poultry, fish or dairy.

Plant-based foods do contain protein, but the proteins in these foods (including grains and legumes) are incomplete. Dr. Mangels explained that proteins are comprised of amino acids. There are nine different amino acids that one's body requires. Animal proteins (meat, fish, dairy, eggs) generally supply ones body with all nine. But each type of plant-based food contains only some of the nine (different plant-based foods contain different amino acids). If your child eats fish, dairy or eggs on a regular basis you don't have to worry about getting enough complete proteins. Otherwise, you need to make sure that your child is eating a wide variety of plant-based foods, so his body gets all nine of the amino acids. In addition, as a vegetarian, your child's body continues to require healthy carbohydrates and fats as well as enough calcium. Strictly vegan children could also become low in B–12, a vitamin important for producing healthy blood and nerves. The table below provides you with suggested foods that will meet your child's nutritional needs.

Nutrients a Healthy Child Needs

Protein: Fruits, vegetables, grains, nuts, nut butters, seeds, legumes, soy products (soy milk, soy beans, soy nuts, tofu, miso, and tempeh), seitan, veggie burgers, and veggie dogs foods containing TVP–textured vegetable protein.

Carbohydrates: Vegetables, fruits, whole grain breads, whole wheat pasta.

Healthy Fats: Nuts, nut butters, legumes, soy products, seeds.

Calcium: Broccoli, bok choy, kale, collard greens, turnip greens, legumes, soy beans, calcium fortified soy or rice milk.

Vitamin B-12: Fortified breakfast cereals (read the label), fortified meat substitutes (e.g., veggie nuggets, burgers, etc.–read the label), nutritional yeast, fortified soy or rice milk.

Vitamin D: Fortified milk, soy milk and rice milk, egg yolks, and fish. Your body also makes it when exposed to sunlight.

Iron: Iron is not absorbed as readily from plant sources as it is from animal sources. So, if your child doesn't eat fish it is important to give your child iron-fortified cereals, breads, rice, and pasta.

Zinc: Yogurt, whole grains, brown rice, legumes, spinach.

As you can see from the table, many foods are in more than one category. It is a good idea to offer these frequently to ensure that your child is getting as wide a variety of nutrients as possible, especially if she doesn't eat fish, eggs or dairy. Remember, don't allow your child to simply replace animal-based proteins with carbohydrates and don't forget to pay attention to serving sizes—they still matter when you're a vegetarian!

❖ ❖ ❖ ❖ ❖

Whether or not your family is vegetarian, helping your child to stretch out or lose weight, certainly takes a little extra effort and planning. Eating out is often when parents find this most challenging. In Chapter Seven, we'll discuss ways that you can continue to help your child eat healthily even when you're not at home.

chapter

Yes! Your Child Can Eat out Healthily

Healthy eating isn't only about what your child eats at home. It's about nutritious eating everywhere and everyday, which, of course, includes eating in restaurants, at the mall, and at the movies. It includes eating fast food, school food, birthday party food, and everything in between. In order for you to help your child achieve great success you have to empower her to be able to eat healthily anywhere and everywhere. This chapter gives you the tools to be able to do just that! It includes a guideline for how to make the best menu choices in a variety of different restaurants and what types of foods to avoid when eating out. You will also find ideas for helping your child eat healthily in many different situations. Happy eating!!

The Basics

As you discovered in the last chapter, it is easy to turn a healthy food into an unhealthy one simply by the way it is prepared. On a restaurant menu, the way an item is prepared usually tells you immediately whether it is a healthy choice for your child. Healthier **Main Menu** foods—those prepared without too much added fat or calories—usually have the following words somewhere in the description: **stir-fried, baked, sautéed in olive oil, grilled, broiled, boiled, roasted** or **steamed.** These are the foods you should consider first when ordering for your child. Of course, portion sizes still count so you should consider asking for an extra plate on the side for sharing or taking home a doggie-bag.

Foods in the **Consume with Care** category are described with words such as **fried, deep-fried, extra crispy, sweet and sour, tempura, extra cheese, hollandaise, creamed, bisque, creamy, rich** or **dense.** It is preferable to avoid ordering these menu items, but if they are favorites, order one as an appetizer for the whole table to share. That way your child (and everyone) gets a taste, without needing to overindulge.

The Details

I want you to be able to take your child to eat in any type of restaurant you choose and, believe it or not, it is possible to be healthy just about everywhere. So, with Dr. Marshel's assistance, I compiled the guide below which you can use every time you take your child out to eat. Don't forget serving sizes and encourage your child to stick to water, seltzer or unsweetened iced tea most of the time.

Pizza

- Choose regular or thin crust type.

- Choose whole wheat crust if it is available (your child probably won't know the difference).

- Good toppings include veggies and chicken. If your child likes salad then "salad pizza"—which is crust and sauce topped with lettuce and other salad ingredients is a great alternative to traditional pizza.

- Don't choose stuffed crusts, extra cheese, beef, pepperoni, sausage or any pizza with the words big, extreme, extra large or supreme in its title.

- Limit the amount of bread and garlic knots that your child eats—better yet, ask the waiter not to bring them to the table.

- One slice equals a serving.

Burgers and Such

- Begin by **not** ordering burgers, sandwiches, fries or other foods whose names contain the following words: super, supreme, big, jumbo, double, mega, ultimate, extreme, deluxe, monster or large. You're really best off choosing items that are small, and perhaps medium for older children.

- Request your child's burger without mayonnaise or any kind of special sauce—which almost always contains mayonnaise. Offer your child a little ketchup for flavor if necessary.

- Offer your child a salad (with light dressing). You may get a strange look the first couple of times, but you'd be surprised to find that many kids really enjoy salad, especially the really plain lettuce and cucumber types that you usually find in a fast food restaurant.

- Milk shakes, thick shakes, or ice cream shakes usually have as many calories and fat as a whole meal. If your child really loves them, get a small one as dessert and split it among at least three people.

- Most burger restaurants now have healthy-choice or "light" sections on their menus. These are not always kid-friendly, but it is definitely worth trying, especially if your child has a slightly more adventurous palate than most.

- Fast-food breakfasts aren't typically fabulous. But if you find yourself there, the best bet for your child is an egg sandwich—it has decent protein and carbohydrate fuel for the day. Hash browns or hotcakes are okay too, but pass on the butter and use only a taste of syrup. I'd suggest you say "no" to the sausage, bacon or biscuits, which tend to be higher in calories and fat and are not as filling or nutritious.

Hot Dogs

- If you can find a low-fat hot dog, go for it.

- Some hot dog restaurants also have food other than hot dogs (like subs or sandwiches), which may be healthier.

- Since hot dogs are typically a high-fat food, it's all about portion size. So, order your child a regular all-beef hot dog, rather than an extra long and stick with a small fries.

- A serving size is one hot dog. If your child is still hungry after one hot dog, offer an ice-pop for dessert rather than a second hot dog.

- Overall, hot dogs are not among the world's healthiest foods. They're packed with artificial flavors, colors, and preservatives. So offer them to your child (at home or out) only once in a while— unless you purchase an all-natural brand.

Chicken

- Order skinless, boneless chicken parts whenever possible, or remove the skin yourself when it is served to your child. Skinless chicken is one of the healthiest, highest protein foods available, especially when ordered *broiled, roasted* or *grilled*. But when chicken is fried (especially extra crispy) or covered with rich sauces it suddenly becomes much less healthy.

- Popcorn chicken and fried chicken nuggets (small pieces of fried chicken) are even less healthy because your child gets less protein and more fat in each mouthful. So choose your child's chicken carefully for a healthy meal.

- As always, say "No" to mayonnaise or other creamy spreads on chicken sandwiches.

Fish and Seafood

- Fried "fish fingers" are a tempting kid-friendly staple at many fish restaurants. But since frying makes very healthy fish much less healthy, it's *much* better to look for broiled or grilled foods and limit fried or battered fish and other seafood.

- Offer your child baked potato (without butter), corn or greens rather than french fries, and order a green salad with light dressing (the more often your order it, the more quickly your child will get used to it!).

- Order fish sandwiches (not fried!) without mayonnaise.

- As with chicken, don't choose popcorn shrimp or fish or fried or battered fish nuggets, fingers or pieces.

Subs and Sandwiches

- Always order a 6-inch sub rather than a footlong for your child.

- If your child likes lettuce, tomato or other fresh veggies, make sure to order them on the sandwich or on the side.

- Offer your child mustard or ketchup, rather than mayonnaise or creamy dressings.

- Offer your child lean meats such as chicken or turkey.

- When possible order a wheat or whole grain, rather than a white roll.

Italian

- If your child enjoys soup, vegetable, minestrone or lentil soups are healthy choices.

- For a main course offer your child chicken marinara, veal marsala, pasta primavera with red sauce (not cream sauce), pasta with red or white clam sauce, pasta fra diablo, fish of the day (broiled or sautéed) or cheese ravioli with marinara sauce (not cream sauce).

- If your child is really stuck, a simple bowl of spaghetti with tomato sauce is fine too.

- Portions still count for all of these! Since Italian restaurants are well-known for overly large portions, the very best way to control for this is to put one portion on your child's plate and then have the rest taken away immediately and put in a bag to be taken home. It would be very helpful to your child if you did the same with your food as well.

- Give your child (and yourself) one piece of bread and then have the bread basket removed from the table, or at least moved away from your side of the table.

Chinese

- Healthy appetizers include steamed vegetable or chicken dumplings or hot and sour wonton or egg-drop soup.

- Good choices for main courses include chicken or fish with Chinese vegetables, chicken or beef with broccoli or mushrooms, chicken or vegetable chow mein, or beef with black bean sauce.

- Have your child avoid fried food.

- Encourage your child to eat brown rather than white rice.

- Don't forget serving sizes.

Japanese

- Miso or vegetable soup is a great start as is edamame (Japanese soy beans—kids love these and they're very high in protein!) or steamed dumplings.

- If you're comfortable with your child eating raw fish, then sushi and sashimi are healthy choices. Otherwise teriyaki and sukiyaki are good options.

- Children often like tempura—a popular Japanese dish. But, this is one to avoid—it involves deep frying vegetables, shrimp, and other foods, which immediately makes these otherwise healthy ingredients into an unhealthy appetizer or meal.

Diners and Family Restaurants

- In a diner offer your child scrambled eggs or an omelet. When you add vegetables to the omelet it becomes even more filling as well as healthier. Some children even prefer an egg-white omelet (my 13-year old son Max has been eating egg-white mushroom omelets since he was about eight years old—it's one of his favorite meals and he doesn't like regular omelets). Eggs usually come with fries or hash browns and toast. Offer your child one or the other and either way limit the choice to at least half or less (e.g., one slice of toast **or** half the order of fries or hash browns). Grilled chicken or fish are also good choices if your child likes them, as is a turkey sandwich.

- Some family-style restaurants have a "low-fat," "low carb," or healthier eating section, which may be a good place to start, if it has any kid-appeal.

- Don't be tempted by kid-friendly menu choices that are fried (like chicken fingers). Also, when ordering from the kids' menu you still need to consider serving sizes.

- Be aware that "diet" meals may not always be as healthy as they seem. This is because they often include portion sizes that are too large. For example, a meal may include a hamburger *and* a very large serving of cottage cheese—that is the equivalent of at least two, maybe three, servings of protein.

- Desserts in some family-style restaurants are usually delicious and enormous, so don't forget to share among many.

- Even better choices for dessert are fruit salad or half a melon.

Steakhouses

- Ask the waiter to recommend the leanest steak possible.

- Choose a small steak for your child.

- You may even consider broiled chicken (remove the skin) or fish, if they're on the menu (only if your child would enjoy either of these as much or better).

- Choose steamed vegetables, such as carrots, broccoli or spinach, and a baked potato (without sour cream) or rice as side dishes (rather than fries or mashed potato). If the potato or serving of rice is large, remove half from your child's plate.

- Order a green salad.

Delicatessen

- For breakfast, instead of a bagel and cream cheese, offer your child scrambled eggs on toast or a roll (whole wheat if it's available).

- Enormous deli muffins are packed with calories. Give your child half a muffin, or even better, only the muffin top.

- For lunch or dinner, chicken breast, sliced turkey, ham or roast beef sandwiches are all good choices—especially on whole wheat bread (mustard or ketchup instead of mayonnaise). If your deli makes extra large sandwiches, give your child half a sandwich or take out some of the meat and save the rest for later.

- Low-fat milk, seltzer or water are the best beverage choices.

- Portion sizes always count!

Sandwich/Soup/Salad/ Stuffed Potato Restaurants

- Pick sandwiches for your child the way you would in a deli—lean meats and poultry with little or no mayonnaise.

- When possible choose whole grain breads, bagels, and rolls, rather than white bread.

- If your child is a soup lover, this can be a healthy choice if you choose right—bean, vegetable, mushroom barley or pea soup are filling and nutritious.

- Offer half a really large baked potato to your child and order it without sour cream and with vegetables.

Mexican

- For soup eaters, black bean soup is a healthy option.

- Healthy kid choices include fajitas; chicken, bean or beef tacos; chicken, bean or beef burritos; chicken, bean or beef enchiladas; or maybe chile con carne if your child is adventurous.

- Mexican food usually comes with healthy black beans.

- It's a good idea to avoid ordering items that include large, fried tortilla shells.

- Ask your server to remove the chip basket from the table after you have served everyone a few chips—this way your child won't be tempted to keep dipping into it and you won't need to be a nag.

- Robyn, one of the parents in my Parents Advisory Group offers a great suggestion. Her family loves salsa, but instead of fried chips, they order it with warm, baked soft tortillas—a sensational substitution!

- Many Mexican dishes arrive covered with melted cheese and sour cream. Ask to have your child's dish prepared with little or no cheese or sour cream.

Greek/Middle Eastern

- Start your child off with hummus (chickpea spread), dolma (stuffed grape leaves), yogurt and cucumber, or avgolemono (lemon) soup.

- Healthy main courses include shish kebab, a chicken gyro or souvlaki or broiled fish.

- Tabouli, couscous (both grains) or rice make a good side dish.

- Always order a salad for your child to try.

- If pita or other bread is on the table, let everyone try a piece and then ask your server to remove it.

- Desserts are gooey, sticky, and sweet—get one or two for the table to share.

Bagel Shops

- If your child will go for it, order whole wheat or other grainy bagels whenever you can.

- Many bagel stores make enormous bagels that equal two or more servings each. In this case, order a mini-bagel or have the inside of your child's bagel scooped out, or give your child half and save the rest for later.

- If your child will *only* eat cream cheese (I know many kids who refuse anything else on a bagel!) use a very thin layer, or use light cream cheese. Do the same for butter.

- If your child will eat other toppings, it is preferable to top the bagel with something nutritious, such as tuna or egg salad (request low-fat mayo), turkey, ham, chicken breast or a scrambled egg.

- If your child's bagel is made with more than a serving of topping you should take some off, ask for a container and take it home for later.

- Bagel stores often sell other goodies, such as croissants, muffins, and other baked goods. Don't let your child tempt you to buy these instead of a healthier choice.

Ice Cream, Frozen Yogurt, and Smoothie Shops

- If you have a choice, choose regular hard or soft-serve ice cream or frozen yogurt over premium hard ice cream.

- Sorbet, ices, and sherbet are even better choices.

- "Premium" ice creams tend to have the highest amount of fat and calories of all. This is because the premium ingredient is cream rather than milk. Premium ice cream is also denser, rather than being pumped with air.

- Toppings add extra calories and fat (especially if the ice cream already has chocolate chips, nuts, etc. inside). Agree to a topping only once in a while.

- A cup is a better choice than a cone (no added calories). A wafer cone is a better choice than a sugar cone. The huge, chocolate-coated sugar cones are the worst choice of all.

- Smoothies made with only juices, low-fat/skim milk, real fruit, and ice are a good alternative to shakes, which should almost always be the last choice for your child.

- Portion control is the key when it comes to frozen treats. Choose a small for your child every single time. Some places even have kids' cups that are even smaller than a small.

Donut and Cookie Shops

- There is no nutritional value in donuts and cookies. But, it's also important to acknowledge the times when your child has a craving for one or is in a situation when everyone else is eating them. In this case your child *should not be deprived*. So, when it comes to these kind of sweets, it's all about how much and how often your child eats them.

- Some donuts and cookies have fewer calories and less fat than others, so don't be afraid to ask for the nutritional information so you can make an educated choice. Of course, your child also has to like the flavor.

- Beware of enormous muffins, crullers, and danishes. A donut, two or three donut holes or a cookie is almost always a better choice.

Convenience Stores and a Quick Stop at the Supermarket

- The best choices at your local market are pretzels, unbuttered popcorn or baked potato chips rather than nachos or fried chips.

- Purchase single size servings for your child, even if they are a bit more expensive. This way there is no temptation to eat more than a serving.

- For a frozen refreshment, a small "slushy," plain fudge bar or fruit juice bar are good choices. Say **No** to the "premium" ice creams that come individually packaged in a box. Kids always seem to go for them.

- In the candy aisle, gum, licorice, hard candy, and mints are much better choices than chocolate bars.

- In the refrigerator, water, flavored water, and seltzer are good choices, rather than soda or other sugar sweetened beverages.

Vending and Vendors

- The best choices are: pretzels, popcorn, baked potato chips, trail mix, nuts, raisins, and sunflower seeds.

School Lunch

- Sending lunch from home gives you the best chance of making sure your child is eating as healthily as possible.

- If your child really wants to eat from the school lunch program, offer it once or twice a week, rather than every day. Get the menu and collaborate with your child to select meals that are the healthiest you can find (this may be a challenge!).

- Talk to your child about eating healthily even when you are not around. Explain that his body will know the difference, whether or not you (or anyone else) is watching. As an example, you might say "You and your body will know if you trade your healthy carrots for someone else's cookies, even if you don't tell anyone else."

Birthday Parties (and any Other Celebration)

- A child should never feel that she is not allowed to eat the food at a birthday party. Therefore, in this case, as in many others, the issue is of portion control.

- *Before* going to each party, remind your child to eat one helping of food and one of dessert and to say "No thank you" to seconds.

- Despite the pre-party discussion, you will most likely need to monitor your child's eating during the party. So, when the pizza comes around, one slice is enough. The same for hot dogs, burgers or any other party meal. When seconds are offered, if necessary gently remind your child that cake or ice cream is still to come. If you are met with "but I'm still hungry," recount by saying, "if you're still hungry after the party, we'll have a healthy snack."

- Since your child has just been to the party, the goodies in the goody bag should be saved for another day (and then perhaps forgotten about and thrown away later by you).

- Many children's birthday parties are "drop-off," making it difficult for you to monitor your child's eating. However, your child's health is more important than her independence. So, for the time being, I'd suggest you either stay at the party to keep a quiet eye on your child or find out when the food will be served (usually near the end) and then come back at that time.

Friends' Homes

- This is one of the most challenging places for an overweight child to try and eat healthily, particularly if the friend is not overweight and junk food is not carefully monitored. It is a battle of will-power that most children are not emotionally equipped to fight, let alone win.

- If your child has typically spent a great deal of time in a neighborhood friend's home where the amount of less healthy food is not carefully monitored, you may need to assess whether this should continue. Perhaps you need to discuss with your child the idea that the time spent with this friend must be in your home with greater frequency. If it is an occasional playdate, it may not be necessary to make any changes.

- Before sending your child to anyone's house to play or for a sleepover, discuss making healthy eating choices while away from home and don't forget the reminder that his body will be affected by what is eaten, whether or not you (or anyone else) is watching.

- It can be frustrating for an overweight child to see thinner friends be able to eat all they want and not gain weight, and this can be even more pronounced when an overweight child enters the home of a friend. It's important to help your child understand and come to terms with this so she doesn't overeat out of frustration. Explain that everyone's body is different and responds to food differently. You can't compare yourself to a friend and you need to do what's right for your body. It's fine to eat some junk food with your friend, but stop after one helping—do what's right for *your* body!

❖ ❖ ❖ ❖ ❖

At this point you have all the information you need to put your child on the road to healthy and nutritious eating. But, I know that sometimes parents worry that you can take healthy eating too far—and what happens if you do? In the next chapter we'll take a look at how to make sure you don't let that happen. I'll also share with you the signs and symptoms of eating disorders—that can strike as young as nine. Keep reading.

Preventing and Understanding Eating Disorders (and Getting Help)

One of the greatest concerns parents express about helping a child lose weight or stretch out is that the focus on *losing weight* can trigger an eating disorder. This is typically more of a concern for parents of girls since the rate of eating disorders among girls is much higher than it is for boys. It is important to note, however, that boys are not immune to eating disorders and if you have a boy who seems to fit any of the risk factors, it is just as important to seek immediate professional help as you would for a girl. So, read this chapter carefully, whether your child is a girl or a boy.

Teaching your child to make healthier eating choices and to exercise—even to lose weight if necessary—is not something that can cause a child to develop an eating disorder. But other factors in a child's environment and life can put a child at risk for developing an eating disorder, and the manner in which a parent speaks to a child about weight and weight loss can impact on the way a child feels about his body. This chapter will help you understand how to avoid the pitfalls that can put your child at risk, and also help you to become aware of the possible signs that indicate that your child may be at risk for, or already developing, an eating disorder.

The Risk Factors

Eating disorders often begin as an attempt to lose weight, but in reality they are much more complex and most people that suffer from eating disorders also struggle with one or more of the following: low self-esteem, social difficulties, loneliness, significant family stress, difficulty expressing feelings, depression, anger, or a history of physical or sexual abuse. Eating disorders sometimes run in families and some research shows that there may be a genetic predisposition to certain types of eating disorders.

If everything else is fine in your child's life, then simply talking sensitively to your child about making healthier food and exercise choices is not enough to trigger an eating disorder. But, if you are concerned that your child may be suffering from *any* of the above risk factors it is **critical** that you seek professional help for your child and perhaps for your family.

Choosing Words That Help, Not Hurt

When you begin talking to your child about a healthier lifestyle, it is important to pick words that are supportive, rather than critical. This will immediately give your child a feeling of positive self-esteem, even though you are saying there is something about your child that needs to change. If you continue to speak like this in all conversations with your child about her weight your child will be well armored against low self esteem. Below are some examples. You can mix and match them and feel free to take them as your own!

Sample #1: I've been thinking that our family needs to get more exercise than we have been and even make some healthier eating choices because we're not doing as great a job as we all could be doing. We're all going to work on it together.

Sample #2: I know you feel that you're the only one in the family that needs to lose weight, and that's hard, but we're (mommy/daddy) working on it with you all the way because we love you and we want your body to be healthy and for you to feel good inside and outside.

Sample #3: Remember yesterday when you had a hard time running during soccer? I could see that you felt sad and a little embarrassed about that. Well, I've been thinking that it's time that we started to help you feel better about yourself and the way to do it is to start making some healthier eating choices that will help your body to feel and look healthier. Then you'll be able to run more easily and feel stronger.

Sample #4: The doctor said it's time to begin eating a bit more healthily and really moving our bodies more than we have been, so we're going to make a plan together for how to do that—we'll do it together, okay?

Sample #5: I know you've been feeling bad about not being able to fit easily into the clothing styles that you really want to wear and this really makes you feel sad. It makes me feel sad too to watch you be this unhappy. I'm going to help you make some changes in your life that will make you feel better about your body. The changes won't happen right away, but you'll see the more we work at it, the better you'll feel.

Sample #6: I'm not sure that this is something you even want to discuss and you may get a little angry with me or even disagree, but it's important for us to talk about it anyway. It's time for you and maybe us as a family to begin making healthier eating and exercise choices. I know it's not easy to think about, but I can see that you're not happy about the way your body feels and looks—even though you don't want to talk about it—and we're going to help you take steps to feel better.

Practice What You Preach

In addition to speaking supportively to your child about making a healthy lifestyle change, it is also important to behave in a way that shows your child that you mean what you say. This means providing plenty of positive feedback for your child's efforts, refraining from criticism, even when it seems she's not trying as hard, and making healthy changes *along with* your child.

It is also important to ensure that other members of your family (especially siblings) do not undermine your child's efforts to make healthy lifestyle changes, and that they do not tease or joke with your child for attempts to exercise that may not be successful or may look clumsy; eating "health" foods like salad; asking questions about the nutritional value of foods; wanting to go food shopping. It is also very, very important that you **not allow** other members of your family to make fun or your child (even as a joke) for being overweight. Studies have shown that children can be negatively affected even into adulthood by negative remarks about their weight or body shape, no matter how brief, even if these remarks are made in an otherwise healthy family setting.

By being aware of as many possible ways to protect your child's self-esteem as he goes through the process of becoming healthier, you will further inoculate your child against the possibility of developing an eating disorder. But, just in case you are still worried, the following section gives you the signs and symptoms of eating disorders. Since early intervention offers the very best chance for cure, it is imperative that you seek professional help if you have even the slightest concern that your child may be exhibiting any signs of any of the disorders described below. Start by speaking to your child's pediatrician. If necessary you may then need to speak to an eating disorders professional and/or have your child evaluated at a clinic or hospital.

I consulted with Dr. Neville Golden, a talented eating disorders specialist and, even better, a really great guy (learn more about him in Appendix Two). He shared the critical signs and symptoms that you need to know in order to recognize each of the eating disorders.

Anorexia Nervosa

Anorexia nervosa is characterized by self-starvation along with significant weight loss, a fear of gaining weight and a distorted sense of how large one's body actually is. Anorexia nervosa is a very serious, potentially life-threatening illness from which recovery can be very difficult if intervention does not happen very early.

The Signs

- Your child eats very little, diets strictly, refuses to eat for long periods of time.

- Your child constantly thinks about how many calories are in everything she eats.

- Your child always thinks he's fat, no matter what he actually looks like or what other people tell him.

- She pretends she's not hungry or seems to convince herself that she's not when she really is.

- He tells lies about eating (for example, he tells you that he's eaten when you know he hasn't).

- She pretends she's eating by moving the food around the plate a lot.

- He exercises for hours a day.

- She avoids being with friends because she doesn't want to be around social eating.

- He's developed food rituals (for example, he eats foods in a certain order, chews excessively).

- She complains of feeling cold all the time.

- You notice his hair is falling out—this may look like thinning or excess hair around the sink or in the hairbrush.

- She complains of feeling bloated and/or being constipated.

Bulimia Nervosa

Bulimics engage in secret cycles of overeating a large amount in a very short amount of time—much more than a person would in a regular meal. The bulimic then resolves the uncomfortable, overfull feeling by purging—usually by vomiting, but sometimes by using laxatives or by excessive exercising. This cycle repeats itself, with varied amounts of frequency from person to person—anywhere from once in a while to several times a day. *Bulimics don't necessarily lose weight the way anorexics do.* So, since there are no obvious signs of their illness and because they are very secretive they may keep their disease well hidden for a long time.

Like anorexia nervosa, bulimia nervosa is dangerous. Vomiting is habit forming and can be very difficult to stop—much like drug or alcohol use it can take over a person's life. So too, the need for food on which to binge becomes a strong drive and bulimics may steal food or money to buy food to feed their habit.

Needless to say, the impact that vomiting can have on a person's body, including on the esophagus, teeth, mouth, and digestive tract can be terrible. Frequent bingeing and purging can also affect one's heart, causing it to beat irregularly—which can kill a person. Any concerns you have about your child, no matter how small, should be shared with your medical professional.

The Signs

- You notice large amounts of food missing in a very short time.

- You find wrappers or empty containers stashed or hidden in your child's room or around the house.

- Your child often goes to the bathroom directly after meals.

- You notice telltale signs of vomiting in the bathroom and no one is ill, or you smell vomit around your child.

- You've found laxatives or diuretics or their wrappers in your child's room or hidden in a place your child thought you wouldn't find them.

- Your child has significant concerns about her weight or shape.

- Your child is exercising excessively, even obsessively

- Your child seems to be withdrawing from friends and/or activities and may seem depressed.

Binge Eating Disorder

Much like bulimics, binge eaters will have frequent episodes of eating very large amounts of food in a short period of time. They will feel out of control while they are eating and then feel guilty after they have finished their binge. Most binge eaters will eat in secret. But unlike bulimics, who will then purge to alleviate the guilt, binge eaters will not purge and will therefore typically gain a significant amount of weight.

❧ ❧ ❧ ❧ ❧

Now that you understand the basics about eating disorders, it is most important to remember that if you have any concern at all that your child may be showing any signs of one, you should immediately seek professional help. I can't stress this enough because early intervention gives a child the greatest chance for successful treatment.

Now, let's move on to the last chapter of your child's successful healthy lifestyle makeover—I'm going to show you how to get your child moving and introduce exercise into your child's everyday life.

Let's Get Moving
(It's Easier Than You Think!)

T his is the last chapter, so begin by breathing a sigh of relief and giving yourself a pat on the back. You've read a lot and if you've been following most or all the suggestions, steps, and advice in the preceding chapters, I am confident that you've already come a very long way toward improving your child's health and weight. Now it's time to talk about exercise.

Exercise Is Essential

We all know how important exercise is for children—we hear about it everyday from doctors, in the news, and in the media. Along with nutrition, exercise is essential for a healthy lifestyle. It helps to develop strong bones, a strong heart and muscles, increased self confidence and self-esteem, and a more positive outlook on life. In addition, exercise can reduce the possibility of type two diabetes, high blood pressure, heart disease, and high cholesterol in your child.

But you may not realize that **physical activity is also critical in order for a child to be successful when trying to lose weight or stretch out.** This is because a child cannot easily lose weight or stretch out by healthy eating alone. It would require eating that is far too restrictive. By incorporating physical activity in addition to the healthy eating changes we've discussed throughout the book, your child will have a much better chance of achieving and keeping a healthy body and along with it a greatly improved body image and self esteem.

The Challenge

Many parents express that getting a child to exercise feels like the most difficult part of the process of creating a healthier lifestyle. This is the reason I purposely put this chapter at the end of the book—by now you have so many tools, it's not going to feel like such a burden! In my experience there are three main reasons that getting a child to exercise is perceived by parents as a hurdle (of course, there may be other reasons too).

1. You dislike exercising, so it's hard to become motivated to get your child to exercise.

2. Your child is resistant to exercising (he dislikes it, feels uncomfortable, embarrassed, doesn't think he's good enough at a sport, etc.) and you can't figure out a way around the resistance.

3. The family schedule is so busy there seems to be no time to fit in exercise.

When you think about it in this way, it *can* seem like an overwhelming task to get your child to exercise, but I'd like to suggest an alternative way of viewing exercise that will make it much easier for you to get your child moving.

I spoke with Sarah Schmitt, a children's sports and fitness specialist, a terrific woman and a mom of two awesome little boys (you can read more about Sarah in Appendix Two), who told me something very interesting and important: *children don't need to exercise in the same way as adults.* She explained that children can learn to love exercise *as long as you make it fun for them.* In fact, for children, exercise can mean playing in a physically active way. When you think about it like this, exercise doesn't have to be difficult or burdensome for your child or, just as importantly, for **YOU**!

This chapter is dedicated to helping you make sure that your child is getting enough exercise, as well as to figuring out how to make it fun for your child and manageable for you. By the time you're done reading you will have a much better idea about how to incorporate physical activity into your child's life.

The Medical Must

Before you begin any new exercise program with your child it is important to make sure that your child is physically healthy and able to engage in all types of activity. This is especially true if your child has not been participating in much physical activity until now. A child that is overweight certainly needs to exercise, but may need to begin slowly and build up gradually. So, before beginning any of the suggestions or the activities recommended in this book or anywhere else, take your child to the pediatrician for a full check-up and get medical clearance for physical activity. Then we're ready to go!

Setting the Scene

As we have already learned from Sarah, our exercise guru, **fun** is the key to success when it comes to getting kids to be physically active. But before we begin take some time to complete the three steps below. Step One is important because it will introduce your child to the idea of becoming more active. Step Two is the easiest of the three steps but take your time completing it, because if you do so thoroughly it will be a time-saver later in the chapter. Step Three will be you and your child's inspiration for the future.

STEP ONE: Talk to Your Child About Becoming More Active

Just as you are helping your child to understand the value of eating healthily, it is as important to make sure he understands the value of physical activity. Conversations with your child should be age appropriate and will most likely need to happen several different times. You should talk about how your whole family will work together to be more active and it is especially important not to blame your child for past or current inactivity or have expectations that your child will have to meet alone. Be clear that you plan to work together and show you mean it by providing encouragement, support, and by being a role model all the way. Below are some examples to get you going. You can mix and match them or use whatever works best with your own child.

- **With your seven year old:** "We need to make sure our bodies get enough moving activities everyday, like at gym in school and outside in the playground and even inside when it's cold. Our family has to work together and really make sure that our bodies are getting enough moving time everyday. We're going to work on getting more than we have been so our bodies can be really, really healthy."

- **With your nine year old:** "Exercise and moving activities will help your body to be really healthy along with the healthy eating we're working on. So we need to work together as a family to make sure that we are all exercising and moving enough. We're going to be making some changes so that we include more moving activities in our lives. It'll be fun and make us all feel really healthy and great!

- **With your eleven year old:** "You've been making excellent eating choices and I'm really proud of you. But for your body to really be healthy, it needs physical activity, which includes really moving and sweating. Lately, your body hasn't been getting enough. We're going to work together as a family to make sure that you and all of us are getting all the activity we need. It will be an adjustment, but we'll feel and look better as we get more active."

STEP TWO: Make a List of the Physical Activities That Your Child Already Enjoys Doing

List every single exercise and physical activity in which your child engages, even if it is only once in a while or very occasionally. Divide the list into three sections.

The first section should include **planned activities,** like team sports, individual sports, dance, and martial arts.

The second should be **unplanned activities,** such as bike-riding, skateboarding, jogging, jump-roping, roller skating, swimming, playing ball, jumping on a trampoline, and playing in the playground or backyard.

The third should include **at home indoor activities,** like using a treadmill/stationary bike/elliptical trainer, hula hooping, and dancing to music.

It is important to take your time to make this list as complete as possible because as we go through the rest of this chapter it will provide you with the basis for all the fun physical activities you will use to really get your child moving.

STEP THREE: Make a Short List of Special Physical Activities That Your Family Would Like to Try

Even if you are generally a sedentary family, it is important to take the time to ask your child about any physical activities that would be really interesting to try. In most cases it is best if this is a goal made as a family and it should be a very short list of one or two physical activities that you would really like to try once you have already been working on your healthy lifestyle for a few months. For example, some families make a goal of going on a spectacular hike together, or a wonderful bike ride. Some make their goal an active family vacation and others plan a weekend sailing or snorkeling.

Marilyn Leonard tells about the Leonard family's inspiration goal:

"Our daughter Harley (11) had always wanted to ice-skate on a frozen pond. She told me that once she was feeling healthy enough to skate without becoming out of breath after a few minutes, she wanted to find a frozen pond and go skating. She also told me (secretly at the time) that she was afraid that she was so heavy she'd break the ice. Well, after six months of healthy eating and really being physically active, Harley was feeling and looking much better. We had to drive a couple of hours north to get to a cold enough area to guarantee frozen ponds in the winter—but we found one and we had an amazing time. We're really proud of Harley and she's really proud of herself too. We've set our next family goal—to hike the Grand Canyon.**"**

As you can see, there are many different options—your goal can be big or small, short or long. You and your child should plan it together. It is important to have a goal toward which you will work. Set a date several months in the future. When you reach your goal, send me an email and tell me about it!

Fact-Finding

The American Heart Association (AHA) recommends that every child should get thirty to sixty minutes of physical activity daily during which the child "works up a sweat" (you can find out more about this recommendation and about the AHA in Appendix Three). At first glance this seems like a tall order, doesn't it? But it is really important for your child to reach *at least* the thirty minute goal, so we need to figure out a way for you to help him reach it.

We'll begin by calculating how much exercise your child is already getting. Grab a piece of paper and we'll do some easy math. Begin by making a chart that includes a column for each day of the week, including weekends. First consider how much physical education (P.E.) your child gets in school. She is likely getting physical activity in gym at least two or three times a week. If your child is one of the really lucky ones, perhaps it's even more. If you don't know, find out how many real minutes and how many days a week your child has gym—mark it down.

Now think about recess. Consider how many minutes a day (that's five, not seven days a week) your child gets for recess and realistically whether or not your child can truly be considered active during this time. If your child is not running, playing ball, climbing, swinging, jumping rope or something similar that makes one sweaty, it doesn't count. If you're not sure, ask your child. If you get a vague answer, it's likely that he is not doing something active enough to be considered exercise, so don't count it. The majority of overweight kids are not active during recess—they tend to be intimidated or afraid to participate in sports or other activities that require a lot of movement, and would prefer to engage in more sedentary behaviors. It's a vicious cycle, of course, the physical activity is just what they need to help them become more self confident and lose weight.

Now let's add to the equation any other exercise in which your child engages. This is the place where you would add any **planned activities** from Step Two (above). Do your best to also estimate how much additional time you can add for the other parts of Step Two (if there are any): **unplanned activities** and **at home indoor activities**. Be honest with yourself (you don't have to show this to anyone—you don't even have to tell me about it!), because it doesn't help your child if you inflate his or her activity level unrealistically for the purpose of this exercise.

By the time you have finished adding up all these areas you should have a clear sense of how much moderate intensity (remember the definition above) physical activity your child is getting.

If, by your calculation, your child is coming close to or meeting the expectation of thirty minutes of exercise a day on **all** or at least **most** days (and you feel confident that you have calculated honestly), congratulations!

It probably means you need to focus most of your energy on the other parts of this book and use this chapter to learn new skills and techniques that you may not have known about.

But, if your calculations show you that your child is exercising less than thirty minutes a day, or is doing so on fewer than most days—or both, you will want to read the rest of this chapter carefully and begin to make some changes. But don't be discouraged. There are many ways to infuse fun movement and activity into your child's life. Don't worry, you won't find most of the changes nearly as difficult as you anticipate. Keep reading and you'll see what I mean.

Getting Creative

The easiest way to get your child moving is to find as many ways as possible to introduce exercise into your child's day in a way that your child will enjoy and that *you* will not find a burden. In addition, you will want to increase the baseline activity level of your child's daily life so that she is engaging in more moving activity and less sedentary activity even during "nonexercising" times. It may take some thought at first to come up with ideas, but once you've found the ones that you and your child enjoy it should be fun and easy. As we go through the rest of this chapter you will see many ideas for both official exercising and for active "nonexercising" activities.

Make Your Child's Everyday Life More Active

Here you will find several ideas for "nonexercising" activities that let you sneak activity into your child's life! This is important because it will help you get your child moving without having to face arguments, resistance or complaints that he doesn't want to exercise. The list below gives you a number of examples and I'm sure you can think of many more of your own. If you come up with any really good ones, email them to me at exercise@kidsonlyweightloss.com, so I can share them with other parents.

The most important suggestion I can make is for you to *be a role model for your child*. So the more physical activity you do with your child and for your child to observe, the more likely it will be that your child will learn how to become more physically active and remain so for a lifetime. Keep this in mind as you read the activities below and all the ideas throughout this chapter.

- Park at the far end of the parking lot (rather than searching for the closest spot) and have a walking race to the door of the store.

- Take the stairs instead of the elevator.

- Instead of driving, walk to neighborhood stores.

- Ivy, one of the parents in my Parents Advisory Group suggested creating hikes for collecting leaves, pinecones, shells or other finds from nature for wonderful art projects.

- Assign regular chores that get your kids moving, like taking out the garbage, vacuuming, or making the bed (I can't guarantee that they won't complain about doing chores!).

- Make a game of more novel household chores that require significant exertion. For example, let's rake a huge pile of leaves and then jump in it, who can pull up the most weeds, which team can shovel their part of the driveway first (don't forget to bend your knees!), let's get soaked while washing the car!

- At home play music that your kids like—you'd be surprised how it will get your kids (and you) dancing and moving.

- Keep a ball and Frisbee in your car so you always have it available at the park or beach for a spontaneous catch.

- Go to the playground. Once there it's hard for a child to resist the swings or climbing equipment.

- Get your child a good quality pedometer to wear. At the end of each day have your child mark on a chart how many steps she took. Begin the next day at zero. The goal is to try and increase the number of steps each day—even if it's only by a couple. If you have more than one child old enough to wear a pedometer, you should get one for each child—whether or not she is overweight.

- Take your child with you when you run errands rather than leaving him home to sit around the house (take with a healthy snack and resist the urge to purchase junk food along the way).

Limit TV and Recreational Computer Time to Less Than Two Hours a Day

I will start this section with a disclaimer—this will not be the fun part of the chapter! You might want to reread Chapter Three to remind you not only about how too much TV and computer time leads to sedentary behavior and therefore weight gain, but also the impact that TV and the Internet can have on the purchasing and consumption of junk food.

It may make sense to talk to your child about limiting TV and computer time during the discussion in which you talk about the importance of exercising (Step One, above). You can explain to your child how the two go together.

If your child watches a lot of TV and/or spends a great deal of time on the computer, you can expect significant resistance (yelling, arguments) when you announce that you are drastically decreasing the amount of TV/computer time allowed. This is to be expected although it will not be easy, especially if you have more than one child—the rule *must* apply for all children, even if only one is overweight. It is your job as a parent to weather the storm and stick to your guns! If you give in to your child's anger, begging or other forms of protest you will be sending your child a powerful message that loud protests will eventually wear you down. Clearly this is not a parenting message that you want to convey—now or in any circumstance.

After you reduce the amount of TV and computer time allowed, it is important to tell your child exactly how much time they will be allowed to have on the TV and computer—be **very** clear about this and follow through everyday, especially in the beginning. Make exceptions only rarely, under special circumstances.

If your child has a TV in his or her bedroom, you might want to consider removing it or disconnecting the cable, except for during agreed upon times. It can be too tempting for a child to stick to the rules when the TV is right there and there is no one on hand to monitor it's use all the time (remember the statistics in Chapter Three). This is true for the computer as well.

Replace TV and Computer Time with Other Activities

When you reduce the amount of time your child sits in front of a screen there will likely be hours of time that had previously been mindlessly occupied that will now need to be filled. It is not reasonable to expect that your child will now automatically know how to fill this time effectively. It is your job to help your child do so. ***Planning*** and ***participation*** are both important.

By *planning* with your child how the extra time will be spent, there will be less time for boredom, frustration, and resentment. Part of this time should be filled with physical activities—throughout this chapter we'll discuss many ways to bring fun movement into your child's daily life. The rest of the time should be spent engaged in board games, creative playing, art and craft projects, exploring fine motor toys, reading, writing, cooking, helping around the house, and anything else that your child enjoys.

Your participation with your child, as well as the participation of any other caregivers is crucial in making sure that this new plan is successful. It is not enough to tell your child to stop watching TV and go and play. You (and other caregivers) need to spend at least some of the time playing and actively participating with your child. Not only does this role model the behaviors you're trying to engender in your child, it also provides your child the support and encouragement needed to make this important change. **Transitioning from being sedentary to being an active person is a significant, life-altering experience. Your child needs as much support as possible. It is your duty to provide this support.**

> ## A Note About Child Care Providers
>
> In order for you and your child to succeed at reducing the amount of sedentary time your child spends it is important to include ALL child care providers—babysitters, housekeepers, grandparents—in understanding and implementing the changes you make. You will need to explain these changes to your child care provider clearly and make sure that each change is understood. Most importantly, you will need to make sure that your child care provider follows through consistently with each one.
>
> In some cases, a babysitter may be resentful about the change because allowing a child to watch a lot of TV is easier work for the babysitter. In other cases, a grandparent may be inclined to give in to a child's begging because he doesn't want to be the bad guy. You need to assess, monitor, and address these issues as they arise. Remember, your child's health is at stake—this is your most important priority.

Scheduled Activity: Thirty Minutes a Day, Five Times a Week

In order to help your child be active as close as possible to thirty minutes a day, most days of the week, you will need to plan activity for your child, rather than just waiting for it to happen. I recommend that your goal should be to plan five days a week of activity and then aim for two days of unplanned activity.

Take a look at the schedule you made (above) and calculate how many days of scheduled activity your child has. If your child has a planned activity two days a week, it means you will need to plan activity at home on three other days. For example, perhaps your child has a one hour karate class on Mondays and a forty-five minute swimming class on Thursdays, you will need to choose three of the remaining five days of the week to plan an activity of at least thirty minutes each day for your child (or family).

Many parents will need to reassess the activities every few months. For example, when soccer season ends, if your child doesn't join another team sport, you will need to replace soccer days with another form of activity. If your child doesn't participate in any planned activities, that's fine—it just means that you'll need to use this chapter to come up with five days of planned activities for your child. I offer you one caveat, be cautious about overscheduling your child. An exhausted child won't have the necessary energy for physical activity, school work or having fun.

Traditional Sports (Outdoor Activities)

If you have a child that enjoys traditional sports (always check back to your list from Step Two) the easiest way to make sure your child gets regular exercise is to schedule in thirty minutes of the sport that your child enjoys. The very best way to do so is to get out there with your child, or have another adult or teenage child care provider do so in your place. Making sure someone reliable supervises is important because otherwise your child may not engage in the activity fully or may not spend a full thirty minutes doing so. If your child is playing with a group of other kids, it may not be appropriate for an adult to be actively involved. However, it is still necessary to keep an eye on your child to make sure that she is really a participant, rather than just an observer.

The easiest sports for kids to play in the backyard, street, driveway or playground are: soccer, tennis (against a wall/garage door), basketball (hoop in driveway), bike riding, roller skating/blading, or skateboarding. Providing lots of positive reinforcement and encouragement throughout the activity will make your child want to continue and do it again. This is not a time to be critical or negative. It is also not a time to make teaching new skills the priority. Simply having fun, moving, and sweating are the main goals.

Of course, it is important to make sure your child wears the appropriate protective equipment for all sports. While some overweight kids resist this because it feels uncomfortable on their bodies, this is not a rule you should bend. Lives are saved and bones are saved every year because children are properly equipped for safety.

In addition to safety equipment, children that exercise need to be well hydrated—with water! Sugar sweetened sports drinks and other sugary beverages should not be offered to your child as a way to quench thirst during or after exercise. Despite what your child may try to tell you, his body does not require the ingredients that sports drinks offer. What's more, the sugar and calories far outweigh any possible gain that these ingredients may have for your child. Sports drinks are marketed to youth, but they are not actually necessary or even good for kids—any more than soda.

If Your Child Dislikes Sports

Some overweight children do not enjoy sports or other typical activities. This is often because they don't feel comfortable or coordinated engaging in these activities. They may feel embarrassed or may have had negative experiences (like always being picked last for a team). Even suggestions to bike ride, skateboard or roller skate might be met with resistance when children find themselves easily out of breath or uncomfortable using the equipment.

If this sounds familiar, it is essential to find at least one activity your child will enjoy. Sometimes practicing privately with your child can help to increase self-confidence as well as your child's skill level. Your child may be thrilled and relieved that you are taking the time to help him work on mastering a sport that seems to come easily to many other kids. Remember to focus on positive reinforcement, encouragement, and small improvements. Remind your child that competition is not nearly as important as working toward your personal best.

You will also need to figure out a way to get your child moving without nagging, yelling, threatening or punishing. Remember, the goal is for physical activity to be fun for your child. If trying to get your child to exercise becomes a battleground between you and your child, then something is not working. It probably means that you haven't yet found an activity that your child enjoys. Remember, this is not your child's fault. Be patient, supportive, and encouraging. Keep talking to your child until you discover an activity that can work. Perhaps it will be walking.

Walking Can Be Fun

Walking is often an ideal activity for an overweight child who dislikes sports. It requires no equipment (except decent shoes) and there is no competition or comparison involved. But, to make the experience of walking as physical activity FUN for your child—a little forethought is necessary.

To begin with, plan thirty minutes of walking for you and your child and decide which days of the week you will do it. Put it on the calendar as you would any scheduled activity. Your child will be excited to have the thirty minutes of time with you—but only if you use it wisely! In order for your child to enjoy the walking time with you here are six helpful tips:

1. Let your child choose the topics of conversation. Listen, comment, and ask questions—keep the conversation going so your child doesn't focus on exercising or begin complaining.

2. Don't criticize your child about *anything* for *any* reason—this isn't the time to be negative.

3. Be supportive and encouraging the entire time.

4. Start slowly, build up gradually—if you begin too fast or too long your child will be discouraged.

5. If your child finds music inspirational, bring it along. Perhaps taking the dog for a walk provides inspiration for your child.

6. Be silly—walk sideways, backwards, skip, hop or gallop along the way—anything to keep the fun and laughter going.

Indoor Activities

Cold or wet weather are not a reason for your child to stop exercising—although these do offer somewhat more of a challenge. In addition, children sometimes need to exercise indoors for other reasons too. Perhaps you have younger children at home with no child care, so you can't simply leave them to take a walk with your older child; maybe you're not feeling well one day and you don't feel like going out to play tennis against the garage; or perhaps you're disabled and unable to stand outside for thirty minutes at a time. These and many other are reasons that developing effective indoor exercising ideas for your child are necessary and important. Without this alternative, your child may end up missing many days of physical activity.

Fitness Equipment

Children as young as eight can use fitness equipment with supervision, as necessary. So, if you have it, this can help you to make sure your child gets thirty minutes of physical activity a day. But, only if your child doesn't find using the equipment boring—this is the complaint I hear most often from kids! The way to almost guarantee that this won't happen is to make sure there is a TV facing the stationary bike/elliptical trainer/treadmill. Tell your child that time watching TV while spent exercising doesn't count towards their TV time. I caution you however to:

1. Limit this time to thirty minutes (if your child isn't tired after thirty minutes see 2).

2. Supervise this time to make sure your child is giving a full effort to exercising while watching TV.

Getting Creative Indoors

Of course, if you don't have exercise equipment, or if your child doesn't like it, you need to find other fun ways to get your child moving indoors. Sarah suggested some really fun games that can also count as physical activity for young kids. In order to make them really effective exercise, don't forget to keep high energy going for a full thirty minutes—you can mix them up to keep it interesting. Also, if necessary, it's fine to split the time into two fifteen-minute exercise periods.

- Duck, duck goose
- Freeze dance
- Tag
- Red light–green light
- Simon says
- "Race against the clock" (I'm timing how long it takes you to get my keys and bring them back to me, etc.)
- Monkey in the middle
- Musical chairs
- Limbo
- Dance Dance Revolution®—this is a video game that simulates the dance game you often see in arcades. In addition to the regular game software, it requires purchasing a dance mat to attach to your game system to be used instead of a joystick. Many kids and parents find this to be a really fun and effective workout.

It's Time for a Commercial Break

Even TV time can be a great opportunity for fun physical activity. In fact, it can be a way to get your child moving and reduce some of the time spent watching commercials. Here's an activity that you can introduce to your family and make your own. It's called **Commercial Break Olympics**. Before the show you are watching begins, select two or three different rooms in your home to be the locations where the different Olympic events will take place. Tell your child what the events will be (they should change each day). Examples include:

- Hopping on one foot
- Push-ups

- Crunches
- Jumping jacks
- Running in place
- Knee bends
- Lunges

Each event lasts two minutes (the length of the commercial break). As soon as the TV segment ends, your child (and you) must run to one of the selected rooms, perform the activity for two minutes and then run back in time for the show to begin again. During the next commercial break, run to a different room and perform a different event. To make this even more fun, you can make up signs that give your child a 10.0 or a 9.5 at the end of each "event." Your child can score your performance as well. If you have more than one child participating, this can be even more fun!

A variation of **Commercial Break Olympics** is to have each participant perform every activity during every commercial break. Pick three rooms in your home and set each one up with one of the activities listed above. Each activity will be performed for a specific number of times. For example, as soon as the segment ends run to a bedroom and do fifteen jumping jacks, then run to the kitchen and hop ten times on each foot, and then lunge back to the TV room.

Of course, **Commercial Break Olympics** can easily be conducted without leaving the TV room at all. Simply turn down the volume of the TV (or turn off the TV for two minutes) and do all the activities right there in place.

Finding Inspiration

For those kids for whom physical activity is an enormous struggle, it's important to keep in mind that they need a constant incentive to keep moving. In order to give your child this incentive, think about what really inspires your child. If your child loves fashion, then perhaps a long walk around the mall, observing all the styles—is a way to sneak in exercise. If your child is creative and artistic, maybe inspirational activity will come in the form of a walk on the beach to collect interesting shells or to observe the sunset that can be recreated later in a painting. If your child enjoys reading, get him age-appropriate books on tape to listen to while exercising.

The Question About Strength Training

For many years there has been great controversy that has swirled around the question of whether children and teens should be able to strength train (lift weights). I spoke to Sarah about this issue, which has of late, been studied by many different experts. She explained to me that it is safe for children to strength train using light weights but only under well supervised conditions to make sure that they use correct form while lifting weights. This is important not only to make sure that they are doing it correctly, but to make sure that they don't injure themselves.

Therefore, I suggest that if you have a local gym, YMCA or JCC that has fitness programs specifically for children, I'd encourage you to enroll your child if this is something that interests your child. However, I'd also strongly suggest that you not allow your child to use weights, or any kind of weight lifting equipment, at home or at a gym without proper supervision from someone trained to work with children and teens (being a parent does **not** count as training in this instance). As a parent you can make sure that your child is getting strength training by including the following types of activities in your child's activity schedule:

- Push ups
- Crunches
- Lunges
- Climbing on the monkey bars
- Knee bends
- A yoga class

Take Another Deep Breath

Congratulations! By now, you're really starting to get your child moving and I bet it's feeling great. Once you find that your child is getting thirty minutes of exercise regularly on most days of the week, you can begin to expand your child's goal to come closer to sixty minutes of physical activity on one or more of those days. You may even find that it's happening naturally.

Now, you're just about at the end of the book. At this point you've crossed the most difficult hurdles of learning. The final pages are about continuing to keep everything you've learned in motion. So turn the page one last time—keeping your energy high and your mind motivated!

The Gift of Health

A s we reach the end of the book I am filled with excitement. If you have read the prior chapters and begun to put into practice the tools, ideas, and suggestions that I have imparted, it means that your child is on the way to having a healthier body, more positive self-esteem, and stronger body image. It also means that your child has a good chance of moving into adulthood as a much healthier person than would have been possible had you not intervened now. This is because there is an excellent possibility that your child will maintain the skills, information, and knowledge that you are beginning to teach and model now, in childhood.

This is very exciting! Each time a parent takes a stand to fight *against* having an overweight or obese child—to fight *for* having a healthy child—it means that this child's risk due to overweight, is lowered for heart disease, diabetes, high cholesterol, high blood pressure, low self-esteem, poor body-image, and social difficulties. This is an incredible and powerful gift that you are able to give your child simply by making the choice to begin taking the steps outlined in the preceding chapters.

You've Just Begun

As you read these last few pages, I want you to think of this not as the end, but as the beginning. I have told you throughout the book that I am with you all the way, but that can only be possible if you continue, *after* you finish reading the book, to follow through will all that you've learned. In order for you to truly gift health to your child, your efforts need to continue for months and years after I've taught you the skills in these pages. So, keep the book with you, reread it in full or review the sections or chapters that are more difficult for you to master. Your child didn't gain weight over-night—it probably took years. So it could take months and even years for you and your child to master a new healthy lifestyle. If your child needs to stretch out, the patience will be in waiting for your child to grow slowly as you introduce healthier eating and exercise. If your child needs to lose weight, this too needs to happen slowly over many months and even years. Rapid weight loss is not healthy for children (it can even be dangerous), nor is it successfully maintained.

Health Equals Love

When you take the time and commit the effort to giving your child the gift of health in a caring, positive, and truly dedicated way, you give your child the consistent message that you love and care very deeply about her entire well being. This feeling will undoubtedly impact positively on your child in many ways. So don't be surprised when your child's self esteem becomes stronger, self-image appears brighter, and relationships with you and others are improved.

The more you invest in your child's health, the more you child will invest in his or her own health. The return on your investment will be huge—it will be greater than you can ever anticipate, more than you ever imagined possible.

I truly mean it when I say that I am with you all the way. I want you to succeed in helping your child to become healthier and happier. I want your child to succeed as well. I would love to hear from you after you have read the book, once you begin making changes and as you, your child, and your family develop a healthier lifestyle. So email me at DrSusan@kidsonlyweightloss.com. I'll be waiting to hear from you and from your child!

Health Is Always First!

DR. SUSAN

Meet the Parents Advisory Group

A s I have told you, I have been fortunate to have a truly dedicated, insightful, intelligent, and incredibly supportive **Parents Advisory Group**. Now I'd like to tell you a little bit more about them. They bring with them an enormous range of experience and come from all different walks of life, backgrounds, ethnicities, and from across the country. Each parent read every single word of the book as I was writing it. Each offered words of advice, critique, suggestions for change, and ideas for additions. They also offered support for me personally along the way. Their thoughts, feelings, and love for their children and teens echo through every page. So too do their hopes that you will take those first steps down the road of health with your child. I thank them from the bottom of my heart for the time and commitment that they gave to me so generously and with such open hearts.

Peter Arango

Peter has been a teacher in independent schools for thirty-six years, and is the former headmaster of a boarding school in Connecticut. He is currently teaching at Cate School in California. He is a storyteller and Shakespeare scholar, a sports fan, and a musician. Peter's wife Mary is also a teacher. In addition she trains therapy dogs and is a nationally known dog photographer. Peter and Mary have three children (31, 19, 15).

Peter remarks, "Our family has come a long way. We do not diet, and we do not restrict, but we do eat thoughtfully and with an eye to health. Information about nutrition has been around for a long time, but as long as we were fighting food, and losing, we couldn't hear what our bodies needed. Giving ourselves permission to eat what we want, in moderation (I eat a piece of dark chocolate every night after dinner for dessert), has quieted all kinds of splurges/urges and has eliminated the binging we used to think of as 'celebration.' "

Keith Benson and Maury Benson

Keith and Maury have been married for twenty-three years. Growing up in Keith's family, food was always the focus at family gatherings. Maury's parents were from the South where the food was fried, more was better, and fat babies meant they were healthier! Maury has struggled with weight her whole life and has educated herself to try and make her family's life healthier. Maury and Keith have three children, two daughters nineteen and sixteen and a son who is eleven. Keith is a pump mechanic who travels frequently for work. Maury works with special needs children and runs a home day care center.

"Our family struggles with healthy eating issues," explains Maury, "we have family history of Type II Diabetes and try to make good choices while on a busy fast paced schedule."

Melinda DiCiro

Melinda is a psychologist who specializes in assessing and helping troubled teenagers and juvenile offenders. Over the past year she has been working at home, researching and writing her own book and taking care of her two daughters, seventeen and fifteen, and her son who is ten. She is married to Nick, an emergency physician. Melinda is an admitted "readaholic," who also enjoys wilderness hiking, traveling, and studying Chinese language and culture. Melinda recognizes that her children will inevitably make their own choices, but that a healthy home base is an effective long term strategy for helping her children's future habits.

"I have come to learn that I am not helpless and without recourse regarding my family's eating habits. I am in charge of what foods I buy and prepare: my taking the time and making the effort to prepare balanced and portion controlled lunches, snacks, and other meals and setting a good example have had a tremendous impact. I recognize that just setting a good example was necessary, but not sufficient!"

Nicole Donoghue

Nicole is a thirty-seven-year-old married mother of a nine-year-old daughter and a six-year-old son. She lives on Long Island, NY and is self-employed as the owner of a property management company. Nicole and her husband, Patrick each have lifelong histories with weight issues. Both suffered from childhood obesity and, as adults, struggle with maintaining a healthy weight. Both Nicole and Patrick come from very tall families as well.

Nicole notes, "It is a fine balancing act to provide healthy options for our family and to let the kids be kids and indulge in the sweets and junk food that bombard them everyday. Our family tries to stay active, which we feel is key to maintaining weight. Both kids are very athletic and play multiple sports. Unfortunately, genetics plays a role and no matter how active and careful we are, we will never be 'tiny, skinny' people. It is important for us to remind both of our children that people come in all shapes and sizes, and the tiny, emaciated role models that flood our home everyday on the

TV and in print are not the norm. A size 4 does not make you better than a size 12."

Judy Jackson

Judy is a single mother of a twenty-one-year-old son and a thirteen-year-old daughter and a grandmother of one little boy. She has been employed by the Northern Arizona Association of Realtors (a professional trade organization with more than 700 members) for fifteen years, eight of these as the Executive Officer. She enjoys travel, reading, and is addicted to crossword puzzles.

Judy acknowledges that she has struggled with her weight her whole life and now sees her daughter facing the same battle. She explains, "As a parent who has struggled with weight and fitness, I feel it is important for me to break the cycle of unhealthy living patterns by exposing my daughter to fitness, health, and good nutrition in order to improve the quality and quantity of her life."

David Larson and Gena Larson

David and Gena are the parents of four children, sons ages fourteen and ten and daughters ages sixteen and eight. Gena teaches language arts at a middle school and enjoys reading, watching sunsets, and spending time with her family. David is the senior pastor of New Life Christian Center in Turlock, CA. He enjoys music, reading, and running. He's run in the Napa Valley Marathon and recently completed his first triathlon. Due to busy schedules, Gena and David struggle to keep fitness and good nutrition in balance within their family—they strive to achieve greater success in these areas. Having a large family has its complexities: three members of their family are slightly overweight and three are not. In addition, some family members are more motivated to engage in physical activity than others. They work to meet everyone's needs each day.

Gena shares that she and David, "desire to raise our children to be compassionate and community involved adults who live balanced and healthy lives."

Robyn Ratcliffe Manzini

Robyn is originally from the Midwest, but she and her husband lived in France for six years where both their children were born. Now in Los Angeles, her family enjoys the outdoors; boating, horseback riding, and hiking whenever they can. Robyn earned an M.B.A. from the University of Chicago and worked for several years in the corporate world. Now, she divides her time between caring for her children and volunteering with the Girl Scouts as a service unit manager for sixty-six local troops, trainer of adult volunteers, troop leader, day camp director, and resident camp program leader. She is on the board of Hill-Harbison House and a member of the DePauw University alumni board. She also volunteers at her children's school and several other charities.

Despite healthy food options, Robyn feels that we live in a world in which sugar and chocolate are ever-present temptations, and that children are challenged with hours spent doing homework with little time left for exercise. Her family is winning the weight battle through patience and open communication about healthy food choices and the need for physical activity. Robyn explains her family's rule which says, "you do *not* have to finish everything on your plate, but you do have to get up off that couch."

Emily Roberts

Emily is a thirty-five year old mother of one daughter, age twelve. She has been married to her husband Jim for fourteen years. She leads a fulfilling and hectic life as a working mom pursuing a rewarding career in retail management. Emily struggled with her weight as a teenager, particularly during the college years. During her early married years she and Jim were at their fittest, but busy lives resulted in their whole family gaining an unhealthy amount of weight over the last several years. After a huge "wake-up call" and a visit to the doctor, Emily and Jim realized that things needed to change, especially for their daughter. They have made some healthy changes over the past year. Emily believes that her daughter has been her inspiration to maintaining their new healthier lifestyle.

Emily speaks of their commitment: "We have been successful at maintaining our healthy lifestyle but realize that we will always have a struggle with weight. We have learned to accept our challenges and deal with them head on; and most importantly we know that with the love and support of each other we can get through anything."

Lois Scaglione

Lois is the mother of two girls, thirteen and eight. For the past twenty-five years she has been working in the insurance industry and eight years ago began working at one of the largest privately held brokerage firms in the United States, handling sports insurance. Growing up, Lois did not struggle with her weight, but recently, as an adult, she has had some challenges in this area and has learned firsthand about making the right food choices to satisfy cravings.

As a mother she began to see her daughters struggling with their weight, so she began educating her family so they would all become healthier and happier. She wants her girls to feel good about themselves and sometimes worries that they focus too much on body image, looking thin and fitting into the latest tight clothing styles. Lois believes that, "establishing proper eating and exercise habits is important since good health and weight maintenance is lifelong."

Jacqueline Schiff and Steve Schiff

Jacqueline and Steve have been married for fifteen years and have a daughter (10) and a son (7). Jacqueline is a clinical psychologist and bases her work in the age old technique of mental imagery, specializing in helping women through challenges of the life cycles. Steve works on Wall Street in the professional derivates market. His career has ranged from computer programming and arbitrage trading to new product development with a passion for economic development and making the banking system more accessible to the world's poor.

Jacqueline explains that their family has gone through many eating styles from macrobiotics and vegetarian to now a more traditional American diet, "We have realized that each family member has different dietary needs. For us the challenge is satisfying each of our needs without having to cook four separate meals. Life is busy and we choose simple, healthy meals."

Ivy Woolf Turk

Ivy is a fifty-year-old divorced mother of a twenty-three-year-old son, nine-teen-year-old daughter, thirty-two-year-old step-son, and thirty-year-old step-daughter. A graduate of Boston University, she lives on Long Island and owns a real estate development firm in New York City. Ivy is also a motivational speaker in homeless shelters in New York City and is writing a book about the experiences of the woman and children in the shelters and their lives and struggles when they leave to reenter the real world on their own.

As a young woman, Ivy struggled with her weight and spent many years learning that using food to push down or avoid feelings was not healthy. As a very busy single, and then blended-family mother, Ivy used food as a way to bring the members of her family together. With her children, Ivy experienced both the struggles of being overweight and the devastation of an eating disorder, after which she found a way to bring the family together around food, but in a healthy way. Ivy began a committed program of healthy eating and exercise, and the kids followed suit. Ivy's daughter Kelly was one of the teens in the **Girls Advisory Group** for *Dr. Susan's Girls-Only Weight Loss Guide: The Easy, Fun Way to Look and Feel Good!* As adults, both daughters and sons are healthy and of normal weight and both sons have gone on to become gourmet cooks. Nowadays, the four adult kids come home from their respective apartments once a month to share a meal. Ivy explains, "It is about a choice to share and love each other and me and express their feelings to each other, both joys and sorrows...and choose to be a family rather than have to be one. The food has become secondary."

Appendix

Meet the Experts

Sarita Dhuper, M.D.

Dr. Sarita Dhuper contributed an enormous amount of medical and nutritional information and expertise throughout the book as well as reading and editing the entire manuscript. She is Clinical Associate Professor of Pediatrics at SUNY Health Science Center of Brooklyn and the Director of Pediatric Cardiology at Brookdale University Hospital and Medical Center in Brooklyn, NY. Apart from her specialty in treating children with congenital heart disease, Dr. Dhuper has been deeply concerned about the rising prevalence of childhood obesity and its associated medical risks. She is Founder and Director of the *Live Light...Live Right* Program, a community based partnership designed to evaluate and treat overweight children with medical risk factors by improving their lifestyle. Dr. Dhuper is a fellow of the American Academy of Pediatrics (FAAP), Fellow of the American College of Cardiology (FACC), and a member of the American Heart Association, The Obesity Society, and American

Obesity Association and serves as a medical consultant for ABC news on childhood obesity.

Dr. Dhuper is married to a physician and has two children. She loves jazz, international travel, and reading philosophy. She believes that in today's society one has to make a special effort to keep children healthy. She firmly believes that "the best medicine is to include an hour of daily physical activity with your child and serve as role models in the daily choices we make."

Neville H. Golden, M.D.

Dr. Neville H. Golden provided his extensive expertise for the eating disorders chapter. He also edited several other chapters. Dr. Golden is co-director of the Eating Disorders Center at Schneider Children's Hospital and Professor of Clinical Pediatrics at Albert Einstein College of Medicine. He is a nationally recognized expert on the medical complications of eating disorders and has published widely on the subject. Dr. Golden lives in Roslyn, NY with his wife, two teenage sons, and a golden retriever. He enjoys hiking, kayaking, and windsurfing. Dr. Golden strongly believes that, "In an otherwise healthy overweight individual, supervised weight loss does not lead to the development of an eating disorder."

Reed Mangels, Ph.D., R.D.

Dr. Reed Mangels contributed all the information about healthy vegetarian eating and edited the section on vegetarian nutrition. She is a nutrition advisor for the nonprofit, educational Vegetarian Resource Group as well as nutrition editor and a regular columnist for the *Vegetarian Journal*, which is published quarterly. She is the coauthor of *Simply Vegan* and *Vegetarian FAQ*.

Dr. Mangels lives in western Massachusetts with her husband, two daughters, and a dog. She has been a vegetarian for about twenty years (vegan for the last fifteen). In a free hour she will read, go for a run with one of her daughters, sew on a quilt or work in the garden. Dr. Mangels' powerful message is to "eat joyfully, mindfully, and compassionately for your own health, the well-being of animals, and the survival of our world."

Judy Marshel, Ph.D., R.D., CD-N

Dr. Judy Marshel contributed her extensive expertise as well as an enormous amount of nutritional information, in addition to reading and editing the entire manuscript. For fourteen years she was the senior nutritionist for Weight Watchers International. Now Dr. Marshel is a nutritionist for the *Live Light. . . Live Right Program* at Brookdale University Hospital and Medical Center, in Brooklyn, NY working with children, teens, and the whole family, to help them move toward their weight and health-related goals. She also has her own health-consulting practice (in Smithtown, Great Neck, and Brooklyn, NY) helping children, teens, and adults to lead healthier lives. Dr. Marshel has also written two books, *Trouble-Free Menopause* and *PMS Relief.*

Dr. Marshel loves to read, spend time with cherished friends, and watch good movies. She also plans to start training for a marathon with a great friend who lives in San Francisco. To achieve optimal health, Dr. Marshel asks us to pay attention to our bodies: "If you are searching for an answer, turn inward. By quieting your mind and listening to your body the wise person inside you emerges and wisdom prevails."

Rebecca Randall, M.S.W.

Rebecca Randall contributed an enormous amount of information, expertise, and experience to Chapter Three. She also read and edited the entire manuscript, not only as an expert, but also with the invaluable eye of a mother. Rebecca is the Director of Outreach at Common Sense Media, the nation's leading nonpartisan, independent organization dedicated to improving the impact of media and entertainment on kids and families. Rebecca graduated magna cum laude from the University of New Hampshire and has an M.A. in Social Service Administration from the University of Chicago. She's been working in the nonprofit sector on behalf of children and families for more than a decade.

Rebecca lives in the San Francisco Bay Area and spends her free time hanging out with her husband and two step-children playing Life, taking walks into town, and having family movie nights. Although her kids are probably sick of hearing about product placement and the use of cartoon characters on food packing, Rebecca continues to explain all the various advertising techniques companies use to get kids to buy their products. Just recently the kids starting pointing out examples to her, so she's decided it might be okay to lay off a bit. Rebecca notes that, "When it comes to our kids' health, what they put into their brains is just as important as what goes into their bodies. So it's vital that kids know how to critically analyze media messages and images."

Sarah Schmitt, M.A.

Sarah Schmitt contributed her expertise on a great deal of information as well as editing the exercise chapter. Sarah is the Sports and Fitness Director at the Sid Jacobson JCC in Roslyn, NY. She oversees the fitness and aquatics departments, the JCC Maccabi Games, and all the adult leagues. Sarah earned a Bachelor's degree in exercise physiology from East Stroudsburg University, where she was a collegiate track and field athlete. She also earned a Master's degree in exercise physiology from Adelphi University. Sarah is a health and fitness instructor with certification from the American College of Sports Medicine and she has been a personal trainer for more than fifteen years.

Sarah is married and has two beautiful sons. Her hobbies include running, cycling, skiing, and horseback riding, but she admits that between having two children under the age of three and working full-time it doesn't leave much time to pursue these very often!

Sarah truly believes that "if we teach children at a young age to have a healthy lifestyle, including good nutrition and exercise, we are giving them the tools to be successful in life."

Appendix

organizations, Websites, Books, and other Useful Information

Resources to Help Your Child Lead a Healthier Life

Alliance for a Healthier Generation
www.HealthierGeneration.org

The Alliance for a Healthier Generation is a joint initiative of the American Heart Association and the William J. Clinton Foundation, with a mission to eliminate childhood obesity and to inspire all young Americans to develop lifelong, healthy habits.

American Heart Association
www.americanheart.org

Increasingly children are at risk for heart disease, stroke, and other cardio-vascular disease. This is why the American Heart Association is working to help kids and families live heart-healthy lives. Visit americanheart.org and click "Children's Health" on the menu on the left-hand side of the page. There are resources for parents and children on topics such as cardiovascular disease, nutrition, physical activity, and childhood obesity. This includes practical tips, such as "How to Limit Tube Time and Get Your Kids Moving" and "How to Get 'Non-Athletes' to Be Physically Active," and the latest scientific statements, such as "Understanding Obesity in Youth" and "Dietary Guidelines for Healthy Children."

The AHA's Scientific Statement that I reference in Chapter Nine which indicates the children need 30-60 minutes of exercise on most days of the week can be found on the AHA website. It is called: *Overweight in Children and Adolescents: Pathophysiology, Consequences, Prevention, and Treatment.* Stephen R. Daniels, M.D., Ph.D.; Donna K. Arnett, Ph.D.; Robert H. Eckel, M.D.; Samuel S. Gidding, M.D.; Laura L. Hayman, Ph.D., R.N.; Shiriki Kumanyika, Ph.D., M.P.H., R.D.; Thomas N. Robinson, M.D., M.P.H.; Barbara J. Scott, R.D., M.P.H.; Sachiko St. Jeor, Ph.D.; Christine L. Williams, M.D., M.P.H. *MPH Circulation.* 2005; 111:1999–2012.

California Project LEAN
(California Department of Health Services)
www.CaliforniaProjectLEAN.org
Tel: (916) 552-9907

California Project LEAN (Leaders Encouraging Activity and Nutrition) has worked with school districts, parents, students, and community leaders to develop and implement policies that support healthy eating and physical activity. Their resources can assist parents who want to get involved in their school community to make changes that make it easier for students to eat healthier and be physically active. I have included Project LEAN as a resource because its website has a great deal of unique and important information and tools for parents no matter where you live.

Common Sense Media

www.commonsensemedia.org

Tel: (415) 863-0600

Common Sense Media is the nation's leading nonpartisan organization dedicated to improving the media lives of kids and families. They provide trustworthy ratings and reviews of media and entertainment based on child development criteria created by leading national experts. Visit them the next time you need help deciding which TV shows, movies, video games, websites, books, or music are most age-appropriate for your kids.

Common Sense provided me with all the statistics and information in Chapter Three. It is a remarkable and very easy to navigate resource for parents—I log on frequently to check out the appropriateness and value of movies, TV shows, and other media for my own three kids.

JCC Association

www.jcca.org

JCC Association is the umbrella organization for the Jewish Community Center Movement, which includes more than 350 JCCs, YM-YWHAs, and campsites in the United States and Canada. JCC Association offers a wide range of services and resources to help its affiliates provide educational, cultural, social, Jewish identity-building, and recreational programs for people of all ages and backgrounds. Among their many and varied resources, JCC's have lead the way in providing services, including a wide range of fitness and wellness programs through sports leagues, clinics, classes, tournaments, and summer camps and facilities for children, teens, and families that develop self-esteem and pride in addition to strong bodies.

Visit www.jcca.org to find your local JCC and other JCC resources.

KidsHealth
www.KidsHealth.org

KidsHealth is one of the largest resources online for medically reviewed health information written for parents, kids, and teens. I find this website to be a tremendous resource, with separate areas for parents, kids, and teens, covering a huge variety of easy to access and understand topics including overweight and obesity.

YMCA
www.ymca.net

The nation's 2,617 YMCAs serve more than 20.2 million people each year, including 9.5 million children, uniting men, women, and children of all ages, faiths, backgrounds, abilities, and income levels. Today with more than 9,000 after school and other programs for youth across the country, YMCAs nationwide are a leading resource for parents looking to find meaningful, fun, and healthy activities for their children. Visit www.ymca.net to find your local YMCA.

Eating Disorders Resources

Eating Disorder Referral and Information Center
www.edreferral.com

The Eating Disorder Referral and Information Center is dedicated to the prevention and treatment of eating disorders. EDReferral.com provides free and treatment resources for all forms of eating disorders. EDReferral. com provides referrals to eating disorder professionals, treatment facilities, support groups, etc. In addition, EDReferral.com provides information for parents on how to deal with a child who has an eating disorder.

National Eating Disorders Association

www.NationalEatingDisorders.org

603 Stewart Street, Suite 803

Seattle, WA 98101

Information and Referral Helpline: (800) 931-2237

The National Eating Disorders Association (NEDA) is the largest not-for-profit organization in the United States working to prevent eating disorders and provide treatment referrals to those suffering from anorexia, bulimia, and binge eating disorders, and those concerned with body image and weight issues. NEDA is dedicated to expanding public understanding and prevention of eating disorders and promoting access to quality treatment for those affected along with support for their families through education, advocacy, and research. In an effort to better support families, the National Eating Disorders Association established the Parent and Family Network (PFN). The PFN is a clearinghouse for up-to-date information about treatment, resources, and advocacy.

Raising a Vegetarian Family

Vegetarian Resource Group

www.vrg.org

P.O. Box 1463, Baltimore, MD 21203

Tel: (410) 366-VEGE [410-366-8343]

VRG is a nonprofit organization that educates the public about vegetarianism, and the interrelated issues of health, nutrition, ecology, ethics, and world hunger. Through the *Vegetarian Journal*, and the website, they provide practical tips for vegetarian meal planning, articles relevant to vegetarian nutrition, recipes, travel and restaurant information, and an opportunity to share ideas with others. They have a List-serv for parents of vegetarian children and brochures and educational tools for children, teens, and parents.

Vegetarian Society of the UK

www.vegsoc.org

This is one of the most popular websites in the UK for vegetarian families, including support for busy parents who want to feed their families well but within a budget. There is even a youth section especially dedicated to younger people who are addressing their diet, packed full of information, tips, and support. I'm recommending this site because even if you don't live in the UK, you'll still find much to learn and enjoy.

VegFamily

VegFamily.com

VegFamily.com is one of the most comprehensive websites dedicated specifically to vegetarian and vegan families. Filled with articles written by leading vegetarian/vegan experts, tips from vegan parents, recipes, interviews, and an "Ask the Dietician" segment to answer nutritional questions, VegFamily helps vegetarian and vegan families deal with everything from being the only vegans at family gatherings to getting enough vitamin B–12.

Books

Moll, L. *The Vegetarian Child: A Complete Guide for Parents.* New York, NY: Perigee, 1997.

Stepaniak, J., and Melina, V. *Raising Vegetarian Children.* New York, NY: Contemporary Books, 2003.

Clothing Resources for Kids Who Are Working on Becoming Healthier

- **Gap** has plus sizes for girls and husky sizes for boys available in stores and online at Gap.com. There is a larger selection available online.

- **Old Navy** has plus sizes for girls and husky sizes for boys in stores and online at OldNavy.com. As with Gap, there is a larger selection available online at OldNavy.com. Between them Old Navy and Gap (both owned by Gap Inc.) have the largest, most varied (style and price) selection of plus size clothing I've seen anywhere!

- **JC Penney** stores and JCPenney.com carry husky boys and plus girls sizes. Some of the parents in my Parents Advisory Group love JC Penney's clothing!

- **Limited Too** and LimitedToo.com, a chain of girls' clothing stores, carries trendy bottoms (pants, shorts, skirts) in half sizes. Several of the parents in my Parents Advisory Group have had great success here.

- **Lands' End** catalog and LandsEnd.com carry girls' plus sizes and boys' husky sizes. Parents in my Advisory Group note that they have particularly terrific bathing suits!

- **Gymboree.com** offers plus sizes for girls and husky sizes for boys up to 10 years old. These sizes are not available at the brick and mortar stores.

❧ ❧ ❧ ❧ ❧

Although this book is not for parents of teens, time flies so quickly that kids become teens before you know it (or perhaps you have a teen at home already). So below are two resources for teenage girls that have been highly recommended by the members of my Parent Advisory Group, so I had to include them!

- **LaneBryant.com** has an online plus size line of clothing called LBmix junior. This line is not available in stores.

- **Torrid** has funky and fashionable clothes that can be purchased either in stores or online at www.Torrid.com.

Index

accessories, 58, 97
advergaming, 46–48
advertising
    Internet/cell phone, 46–48
    in schools, 48–50
    television, 41–43
Alliance for a Healthier Generation,
    190
allowance rules, 50
American Heart Association (AHA),
    161, 190–191
amino acids, 132
anger, 98–101
anorexia nervosa, 153–154
Arango, Peter, 82–83, 180
artificial sweeteners, 110

"baby fat" myth, 15–16, 19–20
babysitters, 167
bagels, 123, 143–144
Benson, Keith, 180
Benson, Maury, 180
beverages
    artificially sweetened, 110
    fruit juice, 114, 119, 124
    healthy choices, 146
    serving sizes, 124
    soda, 110, 114, 124, 146
    sports drinks, 169
    water, 146, 169
binge eating disorder, 155
birthday parties, 147
body image, 51–52, 98
body mass index (BMI), 27–28, 35–36

boys
    body image, 51–52
    eating disorders, 149
    effect of puberty on, 23
breakfast, 76, 120, 123, 136–137, 141
breathing technique, calming, 100
bulimia nervosa, 154–155
bullying, 52–54, 78, 152
burgers, 120–121, 124, 136

calcium, 132
California Project LEAN, 191
calming breathing technique, 100
calorie requirements, 21–22, 111
candy, 146
carbohydrates, 113–115, 131, 132
celebrations, 147
cell phone advertising, 46–48
cereal, 120, 123
Channel One, 49
cheese, 124, 129, 143, 144
chicken, 120, 129, 137–138
child care providers, 167
Chinese restaurants, 139
chips, 124, 125, 128, 143
chocolate, 128, 146
chores, household, 164
Clean Your Plate family pattern, 60–63
clothing
    as negative force, 56–58
    resources, 196–197
    and shame, 95, 96–97
    and sibling stress, 78
Commercial Break Olympics, 172–173

commercials, as negative force, 41–43
Common Sense Media, 41, 47, 192
computer time
    limiting, 80–81, 165–166
    replacing with other activities,
      166–167
Consume with Care foods, 116–117,
    135
convenience stores, 145–146
cookies, 145

Dance Dance Revolution, 172
dancing, 164
delicatessens, 141–142
denial, 30–31
depression in children, 52
desserts, 141, 143
Dhuper, Sarita, 35–36, 115, 116, 128,
    186–187
DiCiro, Melinda, 181
dieting, 21–22, 109
diners, 140–141
divorce guilt, 102, 105
doctor
    check-up before starting exercise,
      158
    child's reaction to, 38–39
    obesity determination myth,
      27–28
    speaking to child about losing
      weight, 37–38
    weight loss recommendation,
      35–36
Donoghue, Nicole, 181–182
donuts, 128, 145

Eating Disorder Referral and
    Information Center, 193
eating disorders, 149–155
    anorexia nervosa, 153–154
    binge eating disorder, 155
    bulimia nervosa, 154–155
    myths, 28–29
    parents as role models, 152–153
    and pressure to be thin, 51
    resources, 193–194
    risk factors, 150

speaking supportively to child,
    150–152
and weighing child at home, 37
eating out, 134–148
    bagel shops, 143–144
    birthday parties/celebrations, 147
    burgers, 136
    chicken, 137–138
    Chinese restaurants, 139
    convenience stores, 145–146
    delicatessens, 141–142
    diners and family restaurants,
      140–141
    donut and cookie shops, 145
    fish and seafood, 138
    food preparation methods, 134–
      135
    friends' homes, 147–148
    giving child options beforehand,
      106–107
    Greek/Middle Eastern restaurants,
      143
    hot dogs, 137
    ice cream, frozen yogurt, and
      smoothie shops, 144–145
    Italian restaurants, 139
    Japanese restaurants, 140
    Mexican restaurants, 142–143
    pizza, 135–136
    sandwich/soup/salad/stuffed
      potato restaurants, 142
    school lunch, 146
    steakhouses, 141
    subs and sandwiches, 138
    vending and vendors, 146
edamame, 140
eggs, 140
Electronics versus Exercise family
    pattern, 79–81
emotional eating, 86–90
errands, running, 165
essential fatty acids, 109
exercise, 156–175
    adding activity to everyday life,
      163–165
    challenge of, 157–158
    check-up before starting, 158

and child care providers, 167
fitness equipment, 171
as fun, 157–158, 169, 173–174
games, 172
goals, 161–163, 167–168
importance of, 156–157
indoor activities, 160, 162, 171–173
limiting TV and computer time,
    165–166
myths, 24
planned activities, 160, 162,
    167–168
replacing TV and computer time
    with other activities, 166–167
setting stage for, 158–161
sports, 168–169
strength training, 174
unplanned activities, 160, 162
walking, 164–165, 170

family
    environment, 23–24
    support, 26–27, 152
    teasing/taunting/name-calling, 78,
        152
family patterns, 59–85
    Clean Your Plate, 60–63
    Electronics versus Exercise, 79–81
    Fast Living, Fast Food, 73–76
    Food Equals Love, 81–85
    Forbidden Foods, 63–67
    overview, 59–60
    Sibling Stress, 76–79
    Snacking is Sweeter, 68–73
family restaurants, 140–141
fashion. See clothing
fast food restaurants, 75, 136–137
Fast Living, Fast Food family pattern,
    73–76
fat-free foods, 109–110, 116
fats, healthy, 115–116, 132
fear, 91–94
feelings about child's weight, 90–107
    anger, 98–101
    fear, 91–94
    frustration, 105–107
    guilt, 101–105

shame, 94–97
fiber, 114
fifteen minute rule, 62, 130
fish, 138
fitness equipment, 171
Food Equals Love family pattern,
    81–85
food labels, 125
food-mood connection, 86–90
foods, 112–119
    Consume with Care, 116–117, 135
    fat-free/nonfat, 109–110, 116
    forbidden, 25–26, 63–67
    fried, 113, 114, 135, 138
    Largely Liquid, 117
    Main Menu, 112–116, 135
    preparation methods, 134–135
    shopping list for, 126–127
    Sweets and Treats, 118–119
    trying new, 117–118
    whole grain, 114, 138, 141–142, 143
forbidden foods, 25–26
Forbidden Foods family pattern,
    63–67
French toast, 120
fried foods, 113, 114, 135, 138
friends, as negative force, 54–55
friends' homes, eating at, 147–148
frozen yogurt. See ice cream/frozen
    yogurt
fruit juice, 114, 119, 124
fruits, 114
frustration, 105–107
fun, physical activity as, 157–158, 169,
    173–174

Gap, 196
genetics myth, 23–24
girls
    body image, 51–52, 98
    eating disorders, 149
    effect of puberty on, 23
Golden, Neville H., 153–155, 187
grandparents, 167
Greek/Middle Eastern restaurants, 143
grilled cheese sandwiches, 129
growing taller, 36–37, 113

guilt, 101–105
Gymboree.com, 196

health benefits to losing weight,
  176–177
healthier life resources, 190–193
healthy eating guidelines, 111–130
  eating enough/no deprivation,
    126–130
  food choices, 112–122
  overview, 111–112
  portion control, 122–125
healthy food choices myth, 18–19
height, in relation to weight, 36–37,
  113
hot dogs, 137

ice cream/frozen yogurt, 124, 128,
  144–145, 146
indoor exercise activities, 160, 162,
  171–173
insulin, 115
Internet advertising, 46–48
iron, 133
Italian restaurants, 139

Jackson, Judy, 182
Japanese restaurants, 140
JCC Association, 192
JC Penney, 196
jealousy, 78
juice, fruit, 114, 119, 124

KidsHealth, 193

Lands' End, 196
LaneBryant.com, 197
Largely Liquid foods, 117
Larson, David, 182
Larson, Gena, 182
laxative abuse, 154, 155
Leonard, Marilyn, 161
licensed merchandise, 44–45
Limited Too, 196

magazines, 51–52
Main Menu foods, 112–116, 135

Mangels, Reed, 131–132, 187–188
Manzini, Robyn Ratcliffe, 143, 183
Marshel, Judy, 113, 119, 123, 135, 188
mayonnaise, 136, 138
media images, as negative force, 51–52
Medical Myths. See myths
Mexican restaurants, 142–143
money, saving, 104
monitoring myth, 27
movies, product placement in, 43–46
movie stars, as negative force, 51–52
muffins, 124, 125, 141, 145
myths, 15–29
  "baby fat," 15–16, 19–20
  dieting, 21–22
  doctor determination of obesity,
    27–28
  eating disorders, 28–29
  exercise, 24
  forbidden food, 25–26
  genetics, 23–24
  healthy food choices, 18–19
  monitoring everything child eats, 27
  puberty, 22–23
  quiz, 16–17
  self-regulation, 20–21
  willpower, 26–27

name-calling, 52–54, 78, 152
National Eating Disorders Association,
  194
Negative Force Factors, 40–58
  ads, 41–43
  fashion, 56–58
  Internet and cell phones, 46–48
  media images, 51–52
  poisonous peers, 52–54
  pressuring peers, 54–55
  product placement in movies/TV,
    43–46
  schools, 48–50
new foods, trying, 117–118
nonfat foods, 109–110, 116

obesity, defined, 27–28
Old Navy, 196
omelets, 140

online shopping for clothes, 57, 78, 96–97, 197–198
Overweight in Children and Adolescents, 191
overweight versus obesity, 28

Parents Advisory Group, 179–185
parties, 147
patience, 177
peanut butter, 123
peanut butter and jelly sandwiches, 120
pediatrician. *See* doctor
pedometers, 164–165
peers, as negative forces, 52–55
physical activity. See exercise
physical education (PE) classes, 24, 162
picky eaters, 129
pizza, 116, 121, 124, 129, 135–136
planned physical activities, 160, 162, 167–168
playgrounds, 164
portion control, 122–125
    birthday parties and other celebrations, 147
    fast food, 75
    frozen treats, 145
    importance of, 26
    Italian restaurants, 139
    serving sizes, 123–125
    snacks, 67, 72–73
potatoes, 115, 123, 142
product placement in movies/TV, 43–46
promotional tie-ins to movies/TV shows, 44–45
protein, 113, 132
puberty, effect on weight, 22–23

quizzes
    Clean Your Plate family pattern, 60
    Electronics versus Exercise family pattern, 79
    facing physical facts, 32–35
    Fast Living, Fast Food family pattern, 73–74
    fear, 92

Food Equals Love family pattern, 81–82
food-mood connection, 87, 88
Forbidden Foods family pattern, 63–64
    Medical Myths, 16–17
    Sibling Stress family pattern, 76–77
    Snacking is Sweeter family pattern, 68

Randall, Rebecca, 41, 45, 188–189
recess, 24, 162
resources, 190–197
    clothing, 196–197
    eating disorders, 193–194
    healthier life, 190–193
    vegetarian diet, 194–195
restaurants. See eating out
Roberts, Emily, 183–184
role models, parents as, 152–153, 164, 166
rules
    allowance, 50
    fifteen minute, 62, 130
    "30 minutes of play time," 80–81
    TV/electronics, 80–81, 165–166

saccharin, 110
salad, 136, 138, 141, 143
salad pizza, 135
sandwiches, 120, 129, 138, 141–142
sandwich/soup/salad/stuffed potato restaurants, 142
sarcasm, 98
Scaglione, Lois, 184
scheduled physical activities, 160, 162, 167–168
Schiff, Jacqueline, 100, 184–185
Schiff, Steve, 184–185
Schmitt, Sarah, 157–158, 171–172, 174, 189
school
    lunches, 146
    as negative force, 48–50
    physical activity during, 24, 162
seafood, 138
seconds, 129–130, 147

self-esteem, 98, 152
self-regulation myth, 20–21
Sensational Substitutions, 119–122,
    128, 143
serving sizes, 123–125. See also
    portion control
shakes, 136, 145
shame, 94–97
shopping
    for clothes, 56–58, 78, 95, 96–97,
    196–197
    for food, 126–127
Sibling Stress family pattern, 76–79
Silver, Hilton, 16
smoothies, 145
Snacking is Sweeter family pattern,
    68–73
snacks
    healthy, 127
    portion control, 67, 72–73
    while watching television, 43
Snapple, 125
soda, 110, 114, 124, 146
soup, 139, 140, 142
sports, 168–169
sports drinks, 169
steakhouses, 141
strength training, 174
stretching out, 36–37, 113
subs, 138
substitutions, healthy, 119–122, 128,
    143
sugar, 25–26, 114, 118–119
Sweet'n Low, 110
Sweets and Treats foods, 118–119

talking to child
    about clothing, 95
    about physical activity, 159–160
    supportively, 150–152
taste tests, blind, 45
teasing, 52–54, 78, 152
television
    ads as negative force, 41–43
    Commercial Break Olympics,
    172–173
    effect on weight, 42
limiting, 80–81, 165–166
product placement in, 43–46
promotional tie-ins, 44–45
replacing with other activities,
    166–167
snacking while watching, 43
stars as negative force, 51–52
while exercising, 171
tempura, 114, 135, 140
"30 minutes of play time" rule, 80–81
Torrid (clothing resource), 197
trying new foods, 117–118
tuna salad sandwiches, 120
Turk, Ivy Woolf, 164, 185

unplanned physical activities, 160, 162

vegetables, 114
vegetarian diet, 130–133, 194–195
Vegetarian Resource Group, 194
Vegetarian Society of the UK, 195
VegFamily, 195
vending machines, 48–49, 146
vitamin B-12, 132, 133
vitamin D, 133
vomiting, 154, 155

walking, 164–165, 170
water, drinking, 146, 169
weighing
    child at home, 37
    yourself in front of child, 93
weight loss decision, 30–39
    denial of problem, 30–31
    getting doctor's opinion, 35–36
    height considerations, 36–37
    letting doctor speak to child, 37–38
    quiz, 32–35
    talking to child after doctor
    meeting, 38–39
whole grain foods, 114, 138, 141–142,
    143
willpower myth, 26–27

YMCA, 193

zinc, 133